Percutaneous Ventricular Support

Editors

HOWARD A. COHEN
JOSE P.S. HENRIQUES

INTERVENTIONAL CARDIOLOGY CLINICS

www.interventional.theclinics.com

Consulting Editors
SAMIN K. SHARMA
IGOR F. PALACIOS

July 2013 • Volume 2 • Number 3

ELSEVIER

1600 John F. Kennedy Boulevard • Suite 1800 • Philadelphia, Pennsylvania, 19103-2899

http://www.theclinics.com

INTERVENTIONAL CARDIOLOGY CLINICS Volume 2, Number 3
July 2013 ISSN 2211-7458, ISBN-13: 978-1-4557-7596-5

Editor: Barbara Cohen-Kligerman

Interventional Cardiology Clinics (ISSN 2211-7458) is published quarterly by Elsevier Inc., 360 Park Avenue South, New York, NY 10010-1710. Months of issue are January, April, July, and October. Subscription prices are USD 188 per year for US individuals, USD 126 per year for US students, USD 281 per year for Canadian individuals, USD 144 per year for Canadian students, USD 281 per year for international individuals, and USD 144 per year for international students. To receive student/resident rate, orders must be accompanied by name of affiliated institution, date of term, and the *signature* of program/residency coordinator on institution letterhead. Orders will be billed at individual rate until proof of status is received. Foreign air speed delivery is included in all *Clinics* subscription prices. All prices are subject to change without notice. **POSTMASTER:** Send address changes to *Interventional Cardiology Clinics*, Elsevier Health Sciences Division, Subscription Customer Service, 3251 Riverport Lane, Maryland Heights, MO 63043. **Customer Service: Telephone: 1-800-654-2452** (U.S. and Canada); **1-314-447-8871** (outside U.S. and Canada). **Fax: 1-314-447-8029. E-mail: journalscustomerservice-usa@elsevier.com** (for print support); **journalsonlinesupport-usa@elsevier.com** (for online support).

Reprints. For copies of 100 or more of articles in this publication, please contact the Commercial Reprints Department, Elsevier Inc., 360 Park Avenue South, New York, NY 10010-1710. Tel.: 212-633-3812; Fax: 212-462-1935; E-mail: reprints@elsevier.com.

Printed and bound by CPI Group (UK) Ltd, Croydon, CR0 4YY

Transferred to digital print 2012

Contributors

CONSULTING EDITORS

SAMIN K. SHARMA, MD, FSCAI, FACC
Director of Clinical Cardiology; Director of
Cardiac Catheterization Laboratory, Mount
Sinai Medical Center, New York, New York

IGOR F. PALACIOS, MD, FSCAI
Director of Interventional Cardiology,
Cardiology Division, Heart Center,
Massachusetts General Hospital; Associate
Professor of Medicine, Harvard Medical
School, Boston, Massachusetts

EDITORS

HOWARD A. COHEN, MD
Professor of Medicine; Director, Temple
Interventional Heart and Vascular Institute;
Director, Cardiac Catheterization Laboratories,
Temple University School of Medicine,
Philadelphia, Pennsylvania

JOSE P.S. HENRIQUES, MD, MBA, PhD
Head of Catheterization Laboratory,
Department of Cardiology, Academic Medical
Center, University of Amsterdam, Amsterdam,
The Netherlands

AUTHORS

YOUSEF H. BADER, MD
Cardiology Fellow, Department of Cardiology,
The Cardiovascular Center, Tufts Medical
Center, Boston, Massachusetts

SUKHDEEP S. BASRA, MD, MPH
Department of Cardiology, Baylor College of
Medicine, Houston, Texas

DANIEL BURKHOFF, MD, PhD
Adjunct Associate Professor of Medicine,
Division of Cardiology, Columbia University in
the City of New York, New York, New York

KIRK N. GARRATT, MSc, MD
Associate Chair, Research and Quality; Director,
Process Improvement and Quality; Director,
Cardiac Interventions; Director, Interventional
Cardiovascular Fellowship Program;
Department of Cardiology, Northshore-LIJ/
Lenox Hill Hospital, New York, New York

IGOR GREGORIC, MD
Department of Cardiology, Center for Advanced
Heart Failure, University of Texas Health
Science Center at Houston, Houston, Texas

RAVI S. HIRA, MD
Department of Cardiology, Baylor College of
Medicine, Houston, Texas

NAVIN K. KAPUR, MD
Assistant Professor of Medicine, The
Cardiovascular Center, Tufts Medical Center,
Boston, Massachusetts

BISWAJIT KAR, MD
Department of Cardiology, Center for
Advanced Heart Failure, University of Texas
Health Science Center at Houston, Houston,
Texas

TIM LOCKIE, MBChB, PhD
Interventional Fellow, Cardiothoracic Centre,
St Thomas' Hospital, Guys and St Thomas'
NHS Trust, London, United Kingdom

PRANAV LOYALKA, MD
Department of Cardiology, Center for
Advanced Heart Failure, University of Texas
Health Science Center at Houston, Houston,
Texas

JUAN N. PULIDO, MD
Assistant Professor of Anesthesiology, Divisions of Cardiovascular Anesthesia and Critical Care Medicine, Department of Anesthesiology, Mayo Clinic, Rochester, Minnesota

SIMON REDWOOD, MD, FRCP, FACC, FSCAI
Professor, Interventional Cardiology, King's College London British Heart Foundation Centre of Excellence, The Rayne Institute, St Thomas' Hospital Campus, London, United Kingdom

CHARANJIT S. RIHAL, MD, FACC
Professor of Medicine and Chair, Division of Cardiovascular Diseases, Department of Medicine, Mayo Clinic, Rochester, Minnesota

TIMOTHY A. SANBORN, MD
Head, Cardiology Division, NorthShore University HealthSystem; Clinical Professor, University of Chicago Pritzker School of Medicine, Evanston, Illinois

HAMMAD SAUDYE, MD
Department of Cardiology, Northshore-LIJ/Lenox Hill Hospital, New York, New York

VEGARD TUSETH, MD, PhD
Department of Heart Disease, Haukeland University Hospital; K2 Department, Institute of Internal Medicine, University of Bergen, Bergen, Norway

RAHUL WADKE, MD
Hospitalist Division, Department of Internal Medicine, Montefiore Medical Center, Bronx, New York

Contents

Cardiogenic shock remains associated with unacceptably high mortality, but recent improvements with early revascularization, continued support with pharmacologic agents, and use of an intra-aortic balloon pump have led to improvements in the rate of mortality. Timely intervention with cardiac surgery in patients with mechanical complications, 3-vessel disease, and left main disease is beneficial. Continued research and ever-improving understanding of this once deadly condition have helped further in improving prognosis. Cutting-edge technologies, such as myocyte cell implantation and the use of a cooling system, will help in pushing the boundaries farther.

Pathophysiologic mechanisms that lead to hemodynamic abnormalities in cardiogenic shock (including hypotension, hypoperfusion, and elevated venous pressures) are reviewed within the framework of pressure-volume analysis. This approach provides the foundation for understanding how different modes of circulatory support impact key these cardiovascular parameters in various clinical settings. Four fundamentally different modes of circulatory support are reviewed, including aortic counterpulsation, left atrial-to-arterial pumping, right atrial-to-arterial pumping, and left ventricular-to-aortic pumping. Each approach has a distinct hemodynamic fingerprint with regard to effects on the ventricular pressure-volume loop and key hemodynamic and metabolic parameters.

Patients who require coronary revascularization and present with poor left ventricular function and complex coronary anatomy are at high risk for percutaneous coronary intervention (PCI) and coronary artery bypass grafting surgery. Some of these patients are poor surgical candidates because of previous cardiac surgery or significant comorbidities. The recent approval and availability of percutaneous left ventricular assist devices has created an opportunity for the highest risk patients. This article reviews currently available mechanical circulatory support systems and portable extracorporeal oxygenation, describing hemodynamic and physiologic rationales, indications, strategies, and available evidence for their use in high risk PCI.

therapeutic options. Hand in hand with innovations in device technology, however, must also come development of integrated circulatory support networks focusing on rapid assessment of patients, multidisciplinary discussion, and timely therapeutic intervention. This article summarizes some of the recent developments in device technology; potential procedures for patient risk stratification, device selection, and response to therapy; management of vascular access to reduce insertion point complications; and some of the expanding potential roles of percutaneous mechanical circulatory support devices.

INTERVENTIONAL CARDIOLOGY CLINICS

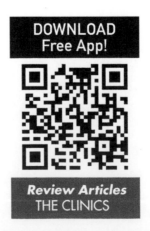

DOWNLOAD
Free App!

Review Articles
THE CLINICS

NOW AVAILABLE FOR YOUR iPhone and iPad

Preface
Percutaneous Mechanical Support

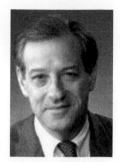

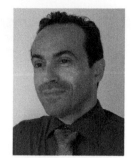

Howard A. Cohen, MD   Jose P.S. Henriques, MD, MBA, PhD
Editors

For more than four decades, intra-aortic balloon counterpulsation has been the initial "go-to" percutaneous device utilized by cardiovascular surgeons and cardiologists for the treatment of cardiogenic shock and to "stabilize" patients with hemodynamic impairment due to myocardial and/or valve dysfunction. The CPS for the percutaneous cardiopulmonary bypass system was utilized briefly but was abandoned due to major systemic complications with any sustained use. A recent meta-analysis and two randomized trials in the setting of acute myocardial infarction and one in the setting of high-risk percutaneous coronary intervention have not revealed a clear benefit of routine usage of the intra-aortic balloon pump (IABP). Although further analyses are still being undertaken, it is clear that these results have put the routine usage of the IABP, and the role of mechanical circulatory support for that matter, in a different perspective.

For approximately the last 10 years, the devices utilized for cardiac support in a variety of scenarios have been expanded to include left atrial to femoral artery bypass (TandemHeart, CardiacAssist, Inc., Pittsburgh, PA, USA) and an axial flow pump left ventricle to ascending aorta (Impella 2.5, Abiomed, Danvers, MA, USA). In addition, an extracorporeal membrane oxygenator has been used in a variety of circumstances as well. These devices provide better circulatory support and superior unloading of the left ventricle, and each has certain advantages and disadvantages.

The purpose of this issue of *Interventional Cardiology Clinics* is to provide the reader with the current "state of the art" in percutaneous mechanical circulatory support describing the background, investigational data, and current concepts in this field as well as a perspective regarding the future of these devices. The authors have been selected because of their particular experience and expertise. The recent IABP story has revealed that the widespread implementation of newer devices needs to be supported by randomized clinical studies and sound evidence. Nevertheless, because of an unmet need, percutaneous mechanical circulatory support devices are finding their way into the clinical arena, and heralding a new era of hope for patients who present with extreme cardiovascular compromise.

Howard A. Cohen, MD
Temple University Hospital
9th Floor Parkinson Pavilion
3401 North Broad Street
Philadelphia, PA 19140, USA

Jose P.S. Henriques, MD, MBA, PhD
Department of Cardiology
Academic Medical Center
University of Amsterdam
Meibergdreef 9
Amsterdam 1105 AZ, The Netherlands

E-mail addresses:
howard.cohen@tuhs.temple.edu (H.A. Cohen)
j.p.henriques@amc.uva.nl (J.P.S. Henriques)

Intervent Cardiol Clin 2 (2013) ix
http://dx.doi.org/10.1016/j.iccl.2013.05.001
2211-7458/13/$ – see front matter © 2013 Published by Elsevier Inc.

interventional.theclinics.com

Cardiogenic Shock
Background, Shock Trial/Registry, Evolving Data, Changing Survival, Best Medical Therapy

Rahul Wadke, MD[a],[*], Timothy A. Sanborn, MD[b]

KEYWORDS

- Cardiogenic shock • Congestive heart failure • Acute myocardial infarction
- Intra-aortic balloon pump

KEY POINTS

- Cardiogenic shock remains associated with unacceptable high mortality, but recent improvements with early revascularization, continued support with pharmacologic agents, and use of intra-aortic balloon pump has led to improvements in rate of mortality.
- Early revascularization with percutaneous coronary intervention is an American College of Cardiology/American Heart Association guideline class I recommendation in patients with cardiogenic shock.
- Timely intervention with cardiac surgery in patients with mechanical complications, 3-vessel disease, and left main disease is beneficial.
- Continued research and ever-improving understanding of this once deadly condition has further helped in improving prognosis. Cutting edge technologies, such as myocyte cell implantation and the use of a cooling system, will help in pushing the boundaries farther.

INTRODUCTION

Shock is a physiologic state characterized by an imbalance between oxygen delivery and oxygen consumption. A prolonged state of oxygen deprivation first leads to cellular hypoxia and cell membrane dysfunction, causing spilling of intracellular contents into extracellular space. Even though the effects of oxygen deprivation can be initially reversible, it can rapidly and irreversibly manifest at a systemic level, leading to end organ damage, multisystem organ failure, and death, and highlighting the importance of rapid recognition and a prompt reversal of shock.

Cardiogenic shock usually results from left ventricular dysfunction in approximately 75% of patients. This pump failure leads to decreased cardiac output and a compensatory increase in the systemic vascular resistance to maintain the perfusion. The diagnosis of cardiogenic shock can be made with the help of hemodynamic parameters gathered from pulmonary artery catheterization. It includes persistent hypotension (systolic blood pressure less than 80–90 mm Hg or mean arterial pressure 30–40 mm Hg lower than baseline) along with severe reduction in cardiac index (less than 1.8 L per minute per meter square without support for less than 2.0 to 2.2 L per minute per meter square) and adequate or elevated filling pressure (left ventricular end diastolic pressure more than 18 mm Hg or right

[a] Hospitalist Division, Department of Internal Medicine, Montefiore Medical Center, 1825 Eastchester Road, Bronx, NY 10461, USA; [b] Head Cardiology Division, NorthShore University HealthSystem, University of Chicago Pritzker School of Medicine, 2650 Ridge Avenue, Walgreen Building, Third Floor, Evanston, IL 60201, USA
* Corresponding author.
E-mail address: rwadke@montefiore.org

Intervent Cardiol Clin 2 (2013) 397–406
http://dx.doi.org/10.1016/j.iccl.2013.03.002
2211-7458/13/$ – see front matter © 2013 Elsevier Inc. All rights reserved.

interventional.theclinics.com

ventricular end diastolic pressure of more than 10–15 mm Hg) (**Table 1**).[1]

Cardiogenic shock remains the most serious complication of acute myocardial infarction (AMI) due to associated extremely high rate of mortality. It is also responsible for most of the deaths associated with AMI. Over the past decade, the 80% to 90% rate of mortality for cardiogenic shock with conservative medical management has shown a significant decrease with early revascularization using percutaneous coronary intervention (PCI) or coronary bypass surgery (CABG).[1–8] At the same time, there is room for improvement in the management strategies to help reduce further the mortality due to cardiogenic shock. The pathologic abnormality of cardiogenic shock is depicted in **Fig. 1**.

INCIDENCE

The incidence of cardiogenic shock had shown remarkable stability over the last few decades.[1–8] Now it appears that with increasing rates of use of primary PCI for an AMI, the incidence of the cardiogenic shock is on the decline.[1,8–10] A longitudinal single community study, with data collected from 1975 and 1997, reported an incidence of 7.1%, while the National Registry of Myocardial Infarction (NRMI),[11] with data collected from 1994 to 1997, reported an incidence of 6.2%.[11] The incidence of cardiogenic shock is approximately twice as high in the setting of ST segment elevation myocardial infarction (STEMI; 5%–8%) as non-ST segment elevation myocardial infarction (2.5%).[1,8–10] The TRACE Registry noted 59% of patients developed cardiogenic shock within the first 48 hours of symptom onset,[12] whereas 10% to 15% of the patients had shock on admission. Early presentation shock has significantly lower 30-day mortality.

CLINICAL PRESENTATION

In addition to signs and symptoms of AMI, patients may present with respiratory difficulties, diaphoresis, and cold and clammy extremities. Signs of end-organ damage may present as oliguria, altered mental status, and severe dyspnea. An S3 gallup on auscultation or a dyskinetic segment of the ventricle may be felt on palpation.

ETIOLOGY

Prior myocardial infarction, older age, female gender, diabetes, hypertension, anterior myocardial infarction, multivessel coronary artery disease, prior diagnosis of heart failure, STEMI, and left bundle branch block have all been identified as risk factors for the development of cardiogenic shock.[1,7–10,12] The most common cause of cardiogenic shock seems to be acute ST elevation myocardial infarction resulting in left ventricular failure. Other causes of cardiogenic shock include extensive right ventricular infarction, ventricular septal rupture, acute severe mitral regurgitation, cardiac tamponade, free wall rupture, aortic dissection, myocarditis, massive pulmonary embolism, and severe valvular stenosis.[1,7–10,12] It is highly critical to recognize these mechanical causes of cardiogenic shock, because different therapeutic options like emergent surgery must be considered for optimal clinical outcome. **Fig. 2** shows the causes of cardiogenic shock.

MANAGEMENT STRATEGIES

Cardiogenic shock is associated with a high rate of mortality. This high rate of mortality has generated an intense interest in developing treatment strategies. Recent improvements in the rate of mortality from cardiogenic shock have been achieved with a better understanding of the disease process, use of a variety of pharmacologic regimens, early revascularization, and use of percutaneous ventricular assist devices.[1,8–10,12]

Recent improvements in mortality and the incidence of cardiogenic shock have coincided with the increased use of intra-aortic balloon pump (IABP) and coronary perfusion strategies.[12] The data from National Registry of Myocardial

Table 1
Heart failure classification

Killip Class/Forrester Classification	Clinical Characteristics	Cardiac Index	Pulmonary Capillary Wedge Pressure
I	No evidence of CHF	>2.2	<18
II	Rales, elevated JVD, S3	>2.2	>18
III	Pulmonary edema	<2.2	<18
IV	Cardiogenic shock	<2.2	>18

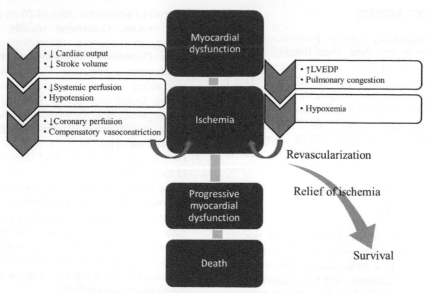

Fig. 1. Pathophysiology of cardiogenic shock. (*Data from* Hasdai D, Topol EJ, Califf RM, et al. Cardiogenic shock complicating acute coronary syndromes. Lancet 2000;356:749–56 and Hochman JS, Buller CE, Sleeper LA, et al. Cardiogenic shock complicating acute myocardial infarction — Etiologies, management and outcome: a report from the SHOCK Trial Registry. Should we emergently revascularize occluded coronaries for cardiogenic shock? J Am Coll Cardiol 2000;36(3 Suppl A):1063–70.)

Infarction (NRMI-2, NRMI-3, NRMI-4) demonstrated decreasing rates of mortality from cardiogenic shock.[11] An American College of Cardiology (ACC)/American Heart Association (AHA) class IIa recommendation is placement of an IABP and class I recommendation of primary percutaneous coronary intervention (PCI) in patients less than 75 years of age.[13,14]

MEDICAL MANAGEMENT

AMI remains the most common cause for cardiogenic shock. The medical therapies being used in the setting of AMI, although not well studied in the setting of cardiogenic shock, remain pertinent to the treatment of cardiogenic shock. The ACC/AHA have outlined guidelines for medical management.[13,14]

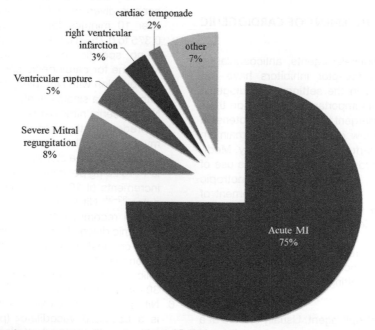

Fig. 2. Causes of cardiogenic shock. (*Data from* Refs.[1,7–10,12])

ANTIPLATELET AGENTS

1. Aspirin irreversibly blocks thromboxane A2 production in platelets, thus helping prevent platelet adhesion after rupture of atherosclerotic plaque. Use of aspirin in ACS is a class I recommendation per ACC/AHA guidelines in patients with unstable angina/non-ST elevation myocardial infarction (NSTEMI)/STEMI.[14–19]
2. Thienopyridines are ADP P2Y12 antagonists that inhibit platelet aggregation. Their use is an ACC/AHA class I recommendation in patients with STEMI.[14,20,21]

ANTICOAGULANTS

Anticoagulants in addition to antiplatelet agents are recommended in the setting of AMI. Unfractionated heparin,[13] low molecular weight heparin, direct thrombin inhibitors, and fondaparinux[22–24] can be chosen depending on clinical picture. There are insufficient data to assess the safety and efficacy of these agents in the setting of the cardiogenic shock. Their use is ACC/AHA class I for STEMI patients undergoing PCI.

GLYCOPROTEIN RECEPTOR INHIBITORS

The glycoprotein IIb/IIIa receptor (GP IIb/IIIa) is one of the final receptors that mediates platelet adhesion and aggregation after plaque rupture.[25–27] Receptor suppression using integrilin therapy (PURSUIT) trial showed no effect on incidence of cardiogenic shock. Their use is ACC/AHA class IIa recommended for STEMI patients.

EMERGENT MANAGEMENT OF CARDIOGENIC SHOCK

Even though antiplatelet agents, anticoagulants, and glycoprotein receptor inhibitors have not been well studied in the setting of cardiogenic shock, they remain important in reperfusion therapy after ACS. Emergent treatment of hypotension and the state of low cardiac output to maintain adequate organ perfusion remain a priority. Medical therapy for cardiogenic shock involves use of sympathomimetic, vasoconstrictor, and inotropic agents. ACC/AHA guidelines for management of cardiogenic shock suggest the use of Norepinephrine. Recent studies have suggested dopamine is associated with a greater number of adverse events when compared with Norepinephrine. However, definitive evidence supporting the use of specific agents in the setting of cardiogenic shock is lacking.

1. Dopamine: inotropic agent. Usually started at a dose of 3 μg per kilogram per minute and slowly titrated to a maximal dose of 20 μg per kilogram per minute. Dopamine usually activates a variety of receptors depending on the dosages. Dopamine has been shown to increase myocardial contractility.[28] Current ACC/AHA guidelines based on expert opinion recommend Dopamine as a first-line agent for cardiogenic shock complicating AMI with moderate hypotension (systolic blood pressure 70–100 mm Hg).[29]
2. Dobutamine: inotropic and vasodilator agent. Dobutamine is very similar in action to dopamine except it is less chronotropic and may decrease afterload. It is usually started at a dose of 2.5 μg per kilogram per minute and can be increased to a maximum dose of 30 μg per kilogram per minute. ACC/AHA guidelines expert opinion does not recommend Dobutamine as a monotherapy in patients with cardiogenic shock.[28,30]
3. Norepinephrine: vasopressor. It is usually started at 2 μg per minute and gradually increased to 20 μg per minute. It is an α-receptor stimulator, used to correct marked hypotension. It is commonly used when cardiogenic shock is not responsive to dopamine.[13] Current ACC/AHA guidelines based on expert opinion recommend Norepinephrine as a preferred agent for cardiogenic shock complicating AMI with severe hypotension (systolic blood pressure less than 70).[29]
4. Milrinone: phosphodiesterase inhibitor. Milrinone lacks adrenergic stimulation and thus has very little effect on myocardia work. Milrinone is given as a 50 μg per kilogram bolus over 10 minutes followed by an infusion of 0.375 to 0.75 μg per kilogram per minute. There is no specific recommendation for use of Milrinone for cardiogenic shock but is used in combination with Norepinephrine or Dopamine rather than a single agent.[30,31]
5. Nitroglycerin: nitric oxide synthase inhibitors. It is predominantly a venodilator, which reduces myocardial wall stress and decreases oxygen requirement. The starting dose for nitroglycerin is 10 to 20 μg per minute and can be titrated by increments of 10 μg per minute every few minutes.[32–35] Nitroglycerine use is an ACC/AHA class I recommendation for relief of ongoing ischemic discomfort or management of pulmonary congestion. Use of nitroglycerine is not recommended in STEMI patients with systolic blood pressure less than 90 mm Hg or 30 mm Hg below baseline.[14]
6. Nitroprusside: nitric oxide synthase inhibitors. It is a balanced vasodilator (preload reduction with venodilation and afterload reduction with

arterial dilation) that reduces myocardial wall stress and decreases oxygen requirement. Nitroprusside is initiated at 5 to 10 µg per kilogram per minute. It can be titrated up to reach a mean arterial pressure goal.[32,33] The use of Nitroprusside is an ACC/AHA class IIa recommendation for no-reflow after PCI, but is not recommended in treatment of cardiogenic shock.[14]

Recommendations for initial reperfusion therapy when cardiogenic shock complicates STEMI are shown in **Fig. 3**. Hemodynamic effects of medications used in cardiogenic shock management are shown in **Table 2**.

MECHANICAL SUPPORT WITH IABP

Without the contraindications of aortic dissection or moderate/severe aortic insufficiency, IABP should be promptly inserted in a patient with cardiogenic shock.[36–53] IABP improves coronary perfusion during diastolic balloon inflation and improves the left ventricular performance during systolic with balloon deflation. IABP can also be placed before revascularization. The NRMI, GUSTO-1, and the SHOCK trial registry have demonstrated reduction in mortality with IABP used in combination with fibrinolysis. Rates of overall and major complications associated with

IABP are 7.2% to 2.8%, respectively. Female gender, small body size, and peripheral vascular disease are the risk factors identified for IABP complications. Placement of an IABP is an ACC/AHA class IIa recommendation in the setting of cardiogenic shock, which is refractory to pharmacologic therapy.[13,14]

EARLY REVASCULARIZATION/REPERFUSION WITH PCI, CABG

The role of thrombolytic therapy has been limited during the era of PCI. Nonetheless, thrombolytics are still used and indicated when PCI is not possible or there is a significant time delay for PCI. Even with a combination of thrombolytics and IABP, rates of mortality continued to be close to 50%, directing the focus to early revascularization.

Several observational studies reported mortality benefits from early revascularization in the setting of cardiogenic shock. In the SHould we emergently revascularize Occluded Coronaries in cardiogenic shocK (SHOCK) trial conducted to understand the effect of early revascularization on the rate of mortality,[1,9,12] 302 patients with STEMI or new left bundle branch block complicated by shock were randomized to either early revascularization strategy (CABG, angioplasty) or initial

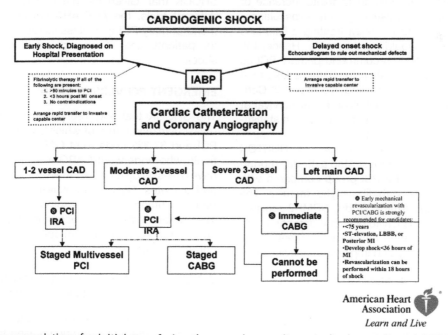

Fig. 3. Recommendations for initial reperfusion therapy when cardiogenic shock complicated STEMI. ACC/AHA 2005 guidelines update for PCI. A report of ACC/AHA task force on practice guidelines 2005. (*Data from* Hochman JS. Cardiogenic shock complicating acute myocardial infarction: expanding the paradigm. Circulation 2003;107:2998–3002.)

Table 2
Hemodynamic effects of medications used in cardiogenic shock management

Medication	Class of Medication	Mechanism of Action	Effects	Dosage
Dopamine	Inotropic	Dose-dependent variable receptors	↑ Contractility, vasoconstriction at high dose	3 µg/kg/min, titrate to max 20 µg/kg/min
Dobutamine	Inotropic, vasodilator	β1 receptors	↑ Contractility, vasodilator	2.5 µg/kg/min, titrate to max 30 µg/kg/min
Norepinephrine	Vasopressor	α receptors	Vasoconstriction	2 µg/min, titrate to max 20 µg/min
Milrinone	Phosphodiesterase inhibitor	↑ Intracellular cAMP	↓ Preload, ↓ afterload, ↑ contractility	50 µg/kg bolus over 10 min, infusion of 0.375–0.75 µg/kg/min
Nitroglycerine	Nitric oxide synthase inhibitor	↑ Intracellular calcium	↓ Preload	10–20 µg/min, increase by 10 µg/min every few minutes
Nitroprusside	Nitric oxide synthase inhibitor	↑ Intracellular calcium	↓ Preload, ↓ afterload	5–10 µg/kg/min, titrate up

medical stabilization and delayed vascularization. Thirty-day survival, 53% for emergency revascularization versus 44% for initial medical stabilization, was not statistically significant ($P = .109$). In 6-month and 12-month follow-up, however, survival differences increased among the 2 groups and reached statistical significance. At the end of the first year there was an absolute increase of 13% in 1-year survival among early revascularization, which essentially meant treating a little less than 8 patients would save one life. Hence, the ACC/AHA guidelines recommend primary PCI as a class 1 recommendation for patients less than 75 years of age with cardiogenic shock.[13] Continued follow-up demonstrated 3-year survival at 38.2% and 6-year survival at 27.6%, both statistically significant ($P = .063$).

Other trials reported similar results. GUSTO-I with 2972 patients demonstrated a 30-day mortality of 30% to 40% for PCI group compared with 60% for patients with fibrinolytic therapy. The Worcester Heart Attack study, NRMI-2 registry, GUSTO-III, and the California state database confirmed the association between emergent revascularization strategy and improved survival.

THE SHOCK TRIAL AND THE SURVIVAL IN ELDERLY

The SHOCK trial survival benefits however did not extend to the subgroup of patients age 75 years or older with AMI and cardiogenic shock.[1,6,12] This subgroup of 56 patients had a 30-day rate of mortality of 75% with early revascularization versus 53% with initial medication management. Other trials with a similar small subset showed mixed results. The Northern New England Cardiovascular Disease Study group had 74 patients aged 75 and older who were enrolled in an early revascularization group. The rate of mortality for this elderly subgroup was 46% compared with 75% in the SHOCK trial. Given the different results among different trials, the ACC/AHA guidelines recommend primary PCI as a class IIa recommendation for patients age 75 or older with cardiogenic shock.

EMERGENT PCI VERSUS CABG

The SHOCK trial had 128 patients in emergent revascularization arm, of which 63.7% underwent PCI and 37.3% underwent CABG.[1,12,50] The patients who underwent CABG were more likely to have 3-vessel disease, left main coronary disease, and diabetes. Despite a relatively worse disease burden, outcome of PCI versus CABG was similar. The authors of the study recommended CABG for consideration as a treatment option with extensive coronary disease.

TREATMENT STRATEGY FOR CARDIOGENIC SHOCK DUE TO MECHANICAL CAUSES

Even though left ventricular dysfunction constitutes by far the most common reason for cardiogenic shock, in 12% of cases, the patient has mechanical complications. These complications include ventricular septal rupture, ventricular free wall rupture, and papillary rupture. Ventricular free wall rupture is associated with 87% rate of mortality. A timely intervention with cardiac surgery is essential for improved survival.[8,54,55]

ADVANCES IN PCI: EMERGENCE OF STENTS, TIMI FLOW, THROMBECTOMY, AND THROMBUS ASPIRATION

The SHOCK trial collected the data in the prestent periods from 1993 to 1994 with 0% stent use and the 1997 to 1998 period with 74% stent use. This change was associated with improved procedural success rate from 67% to 93%.[1,6,12]

TIMI FLOW GRADE SCORING SYSTEM MEASURES POSTPROCEDURE FLOW OF INFARCT-RELATED ARTERY

Studies including the SHOCK trial have demonstrated that low thrombolysis in myocardial infarction (TIMI) flow grades are associated with worsening mortality. Postprocedural TIMI flow score of 3 is associated with 2.3 times higher rate of survival compared with TIMI flow score of 0 to 2.[56–58]

Thrombectomy and thrombus aspiration, not studied in the setting of cardiogenic shock, have shown improvement in reperfusion and reduction in infarct size and rate of mortality. Without more data in patients with cardiogenic shock, its clinical benefit cannot be determined.[59–62]

INNOVATIVE DEVICES AND TECHNIQUES FOR CIRCULATORY SUPPORT

Left ventricular assist devices (LAVDs) and extracorporeal life support are seen as a bridge to cardiac transplantation. The goal of LVAD is to stop the spiraling continued ischemia, allowing time for myocardial recovery, and possibly reversal of neurohormonal imbalances. The device-related complications and irreversible organ failure remain a major obstacle. LVAD essentially circulates oxygenated blood from left ventricle to systemic circulation.

There are 2 devices that have been relatively well studied so far, the TandemHeart PTVA (Cardiac Assists, Inc, Pittsburgh, PA, USA) and Impella Recover LP 2.5 (Abiomed, Inc, Danvers, MA, USA).

The TandemHeart device removes blood from the left atrium and delivers it to femoral artery for a retrograde circulation at a flow rate of 4 L/min. The TandemHeart improves hemodynamic parameters including cardiac index, mean arterial pressure, pulmonary capillary wedge pressure but at the same time, it has been associated with more complications including distal limb ischemia and severe bleeding when compared with IABP.[63–66]

Impella is a device mounted across the aortic valve that can provide a flow rate of 2.5 L/min. The Efficacy Study of LV Assist Device to Treat Patients with Cardiogenic shock (ISAR-SHOCK) trial compared Impella to IABP. The trial had nonclinical outcomes as primary endpoints.[67,68]

Extracorporeal life support involves circulating the blood through the membrane oxygenator, thus not only relieving some workload for the left ventricle but for right ventricle and lungs as well.[69]

SUMMARY

Cardiogenic shock remains associated with unacceptable high mortality. Recent improvements with early revascularization, continued support with pharmacologic agents, and use of IABP has led to improvements in rate of mortality. Early revascularization with PCI is an ACC/AHA guideline class I recommendation in patients with cardiogenic shock. Timely intervention with cardiac surgery in patients with mechanical complications, 3-vessel disease, and left main disease is beneficial. Continued research and ever-improving understanding of this once deadly condition have further helped in improving prognosis. Cutting-edge technologies like myocyte cell implantation and the use of a cooling system will help in pushing the boundaries farther.

REFERENCES

1. Hasdai D, Topol EJ, Califf RM, et al. Cardiogenic shock complicating acute coronary syndromes. Lancet 2000;356:749–56.
2. Goldberg RJ, Gore JM, Alpert JS, et al. Cardiogenic shock after acute myocardial infarction. Incidence and mortality from a community-wide perspective, 1975–1988. N Engl J Med 1991;325:1117.
3. Leor J, Goldbourt U, Reicher-Reiss H, et al. Cardiogenic shock complicating acute myocardial infarction in patients without heart failure on admission: incidence, risk factors, and outcome. SPRINT Study Group. Am J Med 1993;94:265–73.
4. Holmes DR, Bates ER, Kleinman NS, et al. Contemporary reperfusion therapy for cardiogenic shock: the GUSTO-I trial experience. Global utilization of streptokinase and tissue plasminogen activator for occluded coronary arteries. J Am Coll Cardiol 1995;26:668.
5. Hochman JS, Boland J, Sleeper LA, et al, SHOCK Registry Investigators. Current spectrum of cardiogenic shock and effect of early revascularization on

mortality: results of an international registry. Circulation 1995;91:873.

6. Goldberg RJ, Samad NA, Yarzebski J, et al. Temporal trends in cardiogenic shock complicating acute myocardial infarction. N Engl J Med 1999; 340:1162.

7. Hollenberg SM, Kavinsky CJ, Parrillo JE. Cardiogenic shock. Ann Intern Med 1999;131:47.

8. Hochman JS, Buller CE, Sleeper LA, et al. Cardiogenic shock complicating acute myocardial infarction — Etiologies, management and outcome: a report from the SHOCK Trial Registry. Should we emergently revascularize Occluded Coronaries for cardiogenic shocK? J Am Coll Cardiol 2000; 36(3 Suppl A):1063–70.

9. Goldberg RJ, Gore JM, Thompson CA, et al. Recent magnitude of and temporal trends (1997–1997) in the incidence and hospital death rates of cardiogenic shock complicating acute myocardial infarction: the Second National Registry of Myocardial Infarction. Am Heart J 2001;141:65–72.

10. Holmes DR, Berger PB, Hochman JS, et al. Cardiogenic shock in patients with acute ischemic syndromes with and without ST-segment elevation. Circulation 1999;100:2067–73.

11. Babaev A, Frederick PD, Pasta DJ, et al. Trends in management and outcomes of patients with acute myocardial infarction complicated by cardiogenic shock. JAMA 2005;294:448.

12. Hochman JS, Sleeper LA, Webb JG, et al. Early revascularization in acute myocardial infarction complicated by cardiogenic shock. SHOCK Investigators. Should we emergently revascularize occluded coronaries for cardiogenic shock? N Engl J Med 1999;341:625–34.

13. Lindholm MG, Kober L, Boesgaard S, et al. Cardiogenic shock complicating acute myocardial infarction. Eur Heart J 2003;24:258–65.

14. Antman EM, Anbe DT, Armstrong PW, et al. ACC/AHA guidelines for the management of patients with ST-elevation myocardial infarction — Executive summary: a report of the American College of Cardiology/American Heart Association Task Force on Practice Guidelines (Writing Committee to Revise the 1999 Guidelines for the Management of Patients With Acute Myocardial Infarction). Circulation 2004;110:588.

15. Smith SC Jr, Feldman TE, Hirshfeld JW Jr, et al. ACC/AHA/SCAI 2005 guideline update for percutaneous coronary intervention: a report of the American College of Cardiology/American Heart Association Task Force on Practice Guidelines (ACC/AHA/SCAI Writing Committee to Update the 2001 Guidelines for Percutaneous Coronary Intervention). J Am Coll Cardiol 2006;47:e1–121.

16. Anderson JL, Adams CD, Antman EM, et al. ACC/AHA 2007 Guidelines for the Management of Patients With Unstable Angina/Non–ST-Elevation Myocardial Infarction. J Am Coll Cardiol 2007;50: 1–157.

17. Roux S, Christeller S, Lüdin E. Effects of aspirin on coronary reocclusion and recurrent ischemia after thrombolysis: a meta-analysis. J Am Coll Cardiol 1992;19:671–7.

18. Antithrombotic Trialists' Collaboration. Collaborative meta-analysis of randomized trials of antiplatelet therapy for prevention of death, myocardial infarction, and stroke in high risk patients. BMJ 2002;324:71–86.

19. Sagar KA, Smyth MR. A comparative bioavailability study of different aspirin formulations using on-line multidimensional chromatography. J Pharm Biomed Anal 1999;21:383–92.

20. The Clopidogrel In Unstable Angina To Prevent Recurrent Events Trial Investigators. Effects of clopidogrel in addition to aspirin in patients with acute coronary syndromes without ST-segment elevation. N Engl J Med 2001;345:494–502.

21. Sabatine MS, Cannon CP, Gibson CM, et al, CLARITY-TIMI 28 Investigators. Addition of clopidogrel to aspirin and fibrinolytic therapy for myocardial infarction with ST-segment elevation. N Engl J Med 2005;352:1179–89.

22. Antman EM, Morrow DA, McCabe CH, et al. Enoxaparin versus unfractionated heparin with fibrinolysis for ST-elevation myocardial infarction. N Engl J Med 2006;354:1477–88.

23. Stone GW, Witzenbichler B, Guagliumi G, et al. Bivalirudin during primary PCI in acute myocardial infarction. N Engl J Med 2008;358:2218–30.

24. Yusuf S, Mehta SR, Chrolavicius S, et al. Effects of fondaparinux on mortality and reinfarction in patients with acute ST-segment elevation myocardial infarction: the OASIS-6 randomized trial. JAMA 2006;295:1519–30.

25. Coller BS. Platelets and thrombolytic therapy. N Engl J Med 1990;322:33–42.

26. Davì G, Patrono C. Platelet activation and atherothrombosis. N Engl J Med 2007;357:2482–94.

27. Hasdai D, Harrington RA, Hochman JS, et al. Platelet glycoprotein IIb/IIIa blockade and outcome of cardiogenic shock complicating acute coronary syndromes without persistent ST-segment elevation. J Am Coll Cardiol 2000;36:685–92.

28. Leier CV, Heban PT, Huss P, et al. Comparative systemic and regional hemodynamic effects of dopamine and dobutamine in patients with cardiomyopathic heart failure. Circulation 1978;58(3 Pt 1): 466–75.

29. Overgaard C, Dzavik V. Inotropes and vasopressors: review of physiology and clinical use in cardiovascular disease. Circulation 2008;118:1047–56.

30. Bayram M, De Luca L, Massie MB, et al. Reassessment of dobutamine, dopamine, and milrinone in

the management of acute heart failure syndromes. Am J Cardiol 2005;96(6A):47G–58G.

31. Califf RM, Bengtson JR. Cardiogenic shock. N Engl J Med 1994;330:1724–30.

32. Hochman JS. Cardiogenic shock complicating acute myocardial infarction: expanding the paradigm. Circulation 2003;107:2998–3002.

33. Alexander JH, Reynolds HR, Stebbins AL, et al. Effect of tilarginine acetate in patients with acute myocardial infarction and cardiogenic shock: the TRIUMPH randomized controlled trial. JAMA 2007;297:1657–66.

34. Fibrinolytic Therapy Trialists' (FTT) Collaborative Group. Indications for fibrinolytic therapy in suspected acute myocardial infarction: Collaborative overview of early mortality and major morbidity results from all randomized trials of more than 1000 patients. Lancet 1994;343:311.

35. French JK, Feldman HA, Assmann SF, et al. Influence of thrombolytic therapy, with or without intra-aortic balloon counterpulsation on 12-month survival in the SHOCK trial. Am Heart J 2003;146:804.

36. Prewitt RM, Gu S, Schick U, et al. Intraaortic balloon counterpulsation enhances coronary thrombolysis induced by intravenous administration of a thrombolytic agent. J Am Coll Cardiol 1994;23:794.

37. Sanborn TA, Sleeper LA, Bates ER, et al. Impact of thrombolysis, intra-aortic balloon pump counterpulsation, and their combination in cardiogenic shock complicating acute myocardial infarction: a report from the SHOCK Trial Registry. Should we emergently revascularize Occluded Coronaries for cardiogenic shock? J Am Coll Cardiol 2000;36:1123.

38. Anderson RD, Ohman EM, Holmes DR, et al. Use of intraaortic balloon counterpulsation in patients presenting with cardiogenic shock: observations from the GUSTO-I Study. Global Utilization of Streptokinase and TPA for Occluded Coronary Arteries. J Am Coll Cardiol 1997;30:708–15.

39. Barron HV, Every NR, Parsons LS, et al. The use of intra-aortic balloon counterpulsation in patients with cardiogenic shock complicating acute myocardial infarction: data from the National Registry of Myocardial Infarction 2. Am Heart J 2001;141:933.

40. Chen EW, Canto JG, Parsons LS, et al, Investigators in the National Registry of Myocardial Infarction 2. Relation between hospital intra-aortic balloon counterpulsation volume and mortality in acute myocardial infarction complicated by cardiogenic shock. Circulation 2003;108:951–7.

41. Berger PB, Holmes DR, Stebbins AL, et al, GUSTO-I Investigators. Impact of an aggressive invasive catheterization and revascularization strategy on mortality in patients with cardiogenic shock in the Global Utilization of Streptokinase and Tissue Plasminogen Activator for Occluded Coronary Arteries (GUSTO-I) trial. Circulation 1997;96:122.

42. Hasdai D, Holmes DR, Topol EJ, et al. Frequency and clinical outcome of cardiogenic shock during acute myocardial infarction among patients receiving reteplase and alteplase: requests from GUSTO III. Eur Heart J 1999;20:128–35.

43. Edep ME, Brown DL. Effect of early revascularization in mortality from cardiogenic shock complicating acute myocardial infarction in California. Am J Cardiol 2000;85:1185–8.

44. Hochman JS, Sleeper LA, White HD, et al. One-year survival following early revascularization for cardiogenic shock. JAMA 2001;285:190–2.

45. Sleeper LA, Ramanathan K, Picard MH, et al. Functional status and quality of life after emergency revascularization for cardiogenic shock complicating acute myocardial infarction. J Am Coll Cardiol 2005;46:266.

46. Hochman JS, Sleeper LA, Webb JG, et al. Early revascularization and long term survival in cardiogenic shock complicating acute myocardial infarction. JAMA 2006;295:2511–5.

47. Dzavik V, Sleeper LA, Cocke TP, et al. Early revascularization is associated with improved survival in elderly patients with acute myocardial infarction complicated by cardiogenic shock: a report from the Shock Trial Registry. Eur Heart J 2003;24:828–37.

48. Prasad A, Lennon RJ, Rihal CS, et al. Outcomes of elderly patients with cardiogenic shock treated with early percutaneous revascularization. Am Heart J 2004;147:1066–77.

49. Dauerman HL, Ryan TJ, Winthrop WD, et al. Outcomes of percutaneous coronary intervention among elderly patients in cardiogenic shock: a multicenter, decade-long experience. J Invasive Cardiol 2003;15:380–4.

50. White HD, Assmann SF, Sanborn TA, et al. Comparison of percutaneous coronary intervention and coronary artery bypass grafting after acute myocardial infarction complicated by cardiogenic shock: results from the Should We Emergently Revascularize Occluded Coronaries for Cardiogenic Shock (SHOCK) trial. Circulation 2005;112:1992.

51. Stone GW, Marsalese D, Brodie BR, et al. A prospective, randomized evaluation of prophylactic intraaortic balloon counterpulsation in high risk patients with acute myocardial infarction treated with primary angioplasty Second Primary Angioplasty in Myocardial Infarction (PAMI-II) Trial Investigators. J Am Coll Cardiol 1997;29:1459–67.

52. Al Suwaidi J, Berger PB, Holmes DR. Coronary artery stents. JAMA 2000;284:1828–36.

53. Wilson SH, Bell MR, Rihal CS, et al. Infarct reocclusion after primary angioplasty, stent placement and thrombolytic therapy for acute myocardial infarction. Am Heart J 2001;141:704–10.

54. Heuser RR, Maddoux GL, Goss JE, et al. Coronary angioplasty for acute mitral regurgitation due to myocardial infarction. A nonsurgical treatment preserving mitral valve integrity. Ann Intern Med 1987; 107:852–5.

55. Smith EJ, Reitan O, Keeble T, et al. A First-in-man study of the Reitan Catheter Pump for circulatory support in patients undergoing high-risk percutaneous coronary intervention. Catheter Cardiovasc Interv 2009;73:859–65.

56. Chan AW, Chen DP, Bhatt DL, et al. Long-term mortality benefit with the combination of stents and abciximab for cardiogenic shock complicating acute myocardial infarction. Am J Cardiol 2002;89:132–6.

57. Zeymer U, Vogt A, Zahn R, et al. Predictors of in-hospital mortality in 1333 patients with acute myocardial infarction complicated by cardiogenic shock treated with primary percutaneous coronary intervention (PCI): results of the primary PCI registry of the Arbeitsgemeinschaft Leitende Kardiologische Krankenhausärzte (ALKK). Eur Heart J 2004; 25:322–8.

58. Mehta RH, Ou FS, Peterson ED, et al. Clinical significance of post-procedural TIMI flow in patients with cardiogenic shock undergoing primary percutaneous coronary intervention. JACC Cardiovasc Interv 2009;2:56–64.

59. Ikari Y, Sakurada M, Kozuma K, et al. Upfront thrombus aspiration in primary coronary intervention for patients with ST-segment elevation acute myocardial infarction: report of the VAMPIRE (Vacuum aspiration thrombus Removal) trial. JACC Cardiovasc Interv 2008;1:424–31.

60. Svilaas T, Vlaar PJ, van der Horst IC, et al. Thrombus aspiration during primary percutaneous coronary intervention. N Engl J Med 2008;358: 557–67.

61. Sardella G, Mancone M, Bucciarelli-Ducci C, et al. Thrombus aspiration during primary percutaneous coronary intervention improves myocardial reperfusion and reduces infarct size: the EXPIRA (thrombectomy with export catheter in infarct-related artery during primary percutaneous coronary intervention) prospective, randomized trial. J Am Coll Cardiol 2009;53:309–15.

62. Vlaar PJ, Svilaas T, van der Horst IC, et al. Cardiac death and reinfarction after 1 year in the Thrombus Aspiration during Percutaneous coronary intervention in Acute myocardial infarction Study (TAPAS): a 1-year follow-up study. Lancet 2008;371: 1915–20.

63. Thiele H, Lauer B, Hambrecht R, et al. Reversal of cardiogenic shock by percutaneous left atrial-to-femoral arterial bypass assistance. Circulation 2001;104:2917–22.

64. Burkhoff D, O'Neill W, Brunckhorst C, et al. Feasibility study of the use of the TandemHeart percutaneous ventricular assist device for treatment of cardiogenic shock. Catheter Cardiovasc Interv 2006;68:211–7.

65. Thiele H, Sick P, Boudriot E, et al. Randomized comparison of intra-aortic balloon support with a percutaneous left ventricular assist device in patients with revascularized acute myocardial infarction complicated by cardiogenic shock. Eur Heart J 2005;26:1276–83.

66. Raess DH, Weber DM. Impella 2.5. J Cardiovasc Transl Res 2009;2:168–72.

67. Dixon SR, Henriques JP, Mauri L, et al. A Prospective feasibility trial investigating the use of the Impella 2.5 system in patients undergoing high-risk percutaneous coronary intervention (The PROTECT I Trial) initial U.S. experience. JACC Cardiovasc Interv 2009;2:91–6.

68. Seyfarth M, Sibbing D, Bauer I, et al. A randomized clinical trial to evaluate the safety and efficacy of a percutaneous left ventricular assist device versus intra-aortic balloon pumping for treatment of cardiogenic shock caused by myocardial infarction. J Am Coll Cardiol 2008;52:1584–8.

69. Tayara W, Starling RC, Yamani MH, et al. Improved survival after acute myocardial infarction complicated by cardiogenic shock with circulatory support and transplantation: comparing aggressive intervention with conservative treatment. J Heart Lung Transplant 2006;25:504–9.

Hemodynamic Support
Science and Evaluation of the Assisted Circulation with Percutaneous Assist Devices

Daniel Burkhoff, MD, PhD

KEYWORDS

- Circulatory support • Pressure-volume relationships • Pressure-volume area • ESPVR • EDPVR
- Cardiogenic shock • Contractility

KEY POINTS

- Four fundamentally different modes of circulatory support include aortic counterpulsation, left atrial-to-arterial pumping, right atrial-to-arterial pumping, and left ventricular-to-aortic pumping.
- Each approach has a distinct hemodynamic fingerprint with regard to effects on the ventricular pressure-volume loop and key hemodynamic and metabolic parameters.
- An understanding of the different modes of circulatory support may help guide the choice of which device is most appropriate for a given clinical setting.
- Understanding the different modes of circulatory support has the potential to guide future researchers in the optimization of therapies, to help generate hypotheses for clinical trials, and to help guide the choice of device for specific clinical trials that will ultimately provide evidence needed to guide therapeutic decision-making.

INTRODUCTION

The use of percutaneous devices to support the circulation in patients with various forms of hemodynamic compromise and for prophylactic use during high-risk coronary interventions where such compromise is believed likely to occur is becoming more common, which is especially the case as such devices become easier to deploy, safer to use, and hemodynamically more potent. As reviewed in the other articles of this edition, the number of devices and the range of clinical indications in which they are applied are growing. In addition to devices to assist the left ventricle, the value of percutaneous right-ventricular assist devices is becoming increasingly appreciated.

Because different devices have different modes of action, the clinician is faced with the task of choosing the appropriate device for each particular clinical setting. This task can be facilitated by an understanding of the fundamental hemodynamic principles that allow description of the nature and severity of changes in the heart and vascular function in different disease states and the nature and potency with which different devices interact with the heart and vasculature. The goals of cardiac support are different in different settings. For the elective setting of high-risk coronary intervention, the goal is primarily to maintain reasonably normal systemic blood flow and blood pressure during a transient period of coronary occlusion and myocardial dysfunction. In contrast, in more emergent settings, such as cardiogenic shock, pulmonary edema, and pulmonary dysfunction, the goal is often to take over the work, partly or wholly, of the failing right and/or left

Division of Cardiology, Columbia University in the City of New York, 177 Fort Washington Avenue, New York, NY 10032, USA
E-mail address: db59@columbia.edu

Disclosures: D. Burkhoff is an employee of CircuLite Inc, manufacturer of an implantable partial support circulatory assist device. DB has also received educational grant and speaking honoraria from Abiomed.

Intervent Cardiol Clin 2 (2013) 407–416
http://dx.doi.org/10.1016/j.iccl.2013.03.001
2211-7458/13/$ – see front matter © 2013 Elsevier Inc. All rights reserved.

ventricle to ensure normal blood pressure, cardiac output, and pulmonary venous pressures over extended periods of time.[1–5] When these goals are attained, end-organ perfusion and function are maintained, blood can be adequately oxygenated by the lungs, and diuresis is promoted in states of volume overload. Furthermore, by resting the heart and simultaneously ensuring end-organ perfusion in these settings, the odds of native heart recovery without permanent end-organ damage may be improved.

In addition to direct hemodynamic effects, the impact of different devices on coronary blood flow and myocardial oxygen demand can be important, especially in settings of acute coronary syndromes where preservation of myocardial function and viability are of primary concern to maximize the chances of recovery.

FUNDAMENTAL HEMODYNAMIC PRINCIPLES

The ventricular pressure-volume (PV) framework provides a foundation for understanding cardiac and vascular properties, myocardial energetics, and the impact of different modes of percutaneous circulatory support strategies. This framework allows representation of ventricular preload, afterload, lusitropy, and contractility and their respective roles in determining cardiac output, blood pressure, and pulmonary venous pressures. Details of this approach have been summarized previously[6,7] and are reviewed here in brief. The basic concepts are summarized by the pressure-volume relations displayed in **Fig. 1**. (Note that this and all other figures and quantitative values presented in this article have been derived from a previously described and validated real-time, interactive cardiovascular simulation.[8]) The normal PV loop (shown in blue) is a plot of instantaneous ventricular pressure and volume throughout the cardiac cycle. The 4 major phases of the cardiac cycle are readily identified. Starting at end-diastole (bottom right corner), these phases are as follows: isovolumic contraction, ejection, isovolumic relaxation, and filling. The PV loop is bounded inferiorly by the end-diastolic pressure-volume relationship (EDPVR) and superiorly by the end-systolic pressure-volume relationship (ESPVR). The EDPVR uniquely defines the passive diastolic properties of the LV and the slope (E_{es}) and volume axis intercept of the ESPVR provide a load-independent index of ventricular contractility.

In this construct, ventricular preload is indexed by either end-diastolic volume (EDV) or end-diastolic pressure (EDP). Ventricular afterload is indexed by effective arterial elastance (Ea), which is the slope of the line connecting the point on the

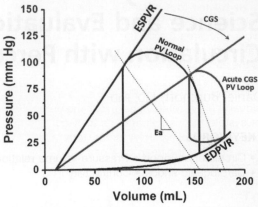

Fig. 1. Prototypical pressure-volume (PV) loops from a normal adult (*blue*) and from a patient in cardiogenic shock (CGS, shown in *red*). The loops are bound by the end-systolic and end-diastolic pressure-volume relations (ESPVR and EDPVR, respectively). The downward shift of the ESPVR is a reflection of the reduction in left ventricular contractility that underlies the development of CGS. Effective arterial elastance (Ea), an index of ventricular afterload, which depends primarily on total peripheral resistance and heart rate, can also be derived from the loop. See text for further details.

volume axis at the EDV to the end-systolic PV point. Ea is mainly determined by total peripheral arterial resistance (TPR) and the duration of the cardiac cycle (T) according to Ea ≡ TPR/T.[9]

One additional hemodynamic parameter of interest is cardiac power output (CPO), which is defined as the product of stroke work (SW, the area inside the PV loop) and heart rate (HR). However, because it is not possible to precisely quantify SW noninvasively, SW is approximated as the product of mean arterial pressure (MAP) and stroke volume (SV). Accordingly, CPO ≡ SW × HR ≈ MAP × SV × HR = MAP × CO. This parameter integrates information related to 2 fundamental functions of the heart: its ability to generate blood pressure and its ability to generate cardiac output. In addition, interest in this parameter has stemmed largely from the fact that for patients presenting with cardiogenic shock (CGS), CPO has an inverse relation to in-hospital and short term survival.[10–12]

Myocardial Oxygen Demand and Supply

Many clinicians think that myocardial oxygen consumption is related to SW (on a per beat basis) or to CPO (on a per unit time basis). However, this is not the case because SW does not quantify all of the work done by the heart with each contraction. Myocardial oxygen consumption has been shown to be related to a parameter called the pressure-volume area (PVA), which is the sum of stroke work (the area inside the PV loop) and what is called the end-systolic potential area (PE).[13] PE is the area contained within the boundary defined by the ESPVR, the EDPVR, and the diastolic portion of the PV loop (**Fig. 2A**) and represents residual energy stored in the myofilaments at the end of systole that is liberated as heat during cross-bridge uncoupling. PVA is the total mechanical work done by the heart on a beat and is therefore closely related to myocardial oxygen consumption: PVA = SW + PE.[14–16] The 5 PV loops shown in **Fig. 2B** are derived with a constant ventricular contractile state but with different values of total peripheral resistance. **Fig. 2C** shows the relationship between myocardial oxygen consumption (MVO_2) for each of the loops as a function of the respective PVA values. When ventricular contractility is increased, the MVO_2-PVA relationship shifts upward in a parallel manner; conversely, when contractility decreases, the MOV_2-PVA relationship shifts downward in a parallel manner.[14] Because PVA relates to oxygen consumption per beat, it should be appreciated that the heart rate is a potent modulator of oxygen consumption per unit of time, because oxygen consumption per minute will be related to PVA × HR.

Oxygen is provided to the myocardium by blood delivered through the coronary arteries and microcirculation. Under normal conditions, the heart extracts more oxygen from blood than any other organ in the body, capable of attaining arterial-venous oxygen content differences of more than 15 mL O_2/100 mL blood, with typical arterial oxygen content of 20 mL O_2/100 mL blood. In addition, unlike other organs, the heart relies nearly completely on aerobic metabolism, necessitating oxygen to sustain myocardial contraction. Therefore, under conditions of increased myocardial oxygen demand, there must be increased blood flow to maintain increased levels of total mechanical work. Coronary blood flow is regulated by metabolic, neural, humoral, autoregulatory, extravascular compressive, and diastolic phase-related factors.[17,18] If coronary blood flow cannot increase to meet myocardial needs, increased workloads cannot be sustained. Similarly, when blood flow is limited (eg, by pathologic coronary occlusion by a thrombus or by occlusion during percutaneous intervention), myocardial workload decreases in an attempt to balance oxygen supply and demand. In general, the mechanism of reducing workload is accomplished by auto-downregulation of myocardial contractility in the affected (ischemic) region. If such a balance cannot be attained, myocardial necrosis ensues within short periods of time (eg, on the order of 10 min).

If heart rate and epicardial resistance are fixed, as occurs with severe (although not total) coronary occlusion, blood flow can be increased mainly by either augmenting MAP, or by decreasing right atrial or LV end-diastolic pressure. Thus, in some

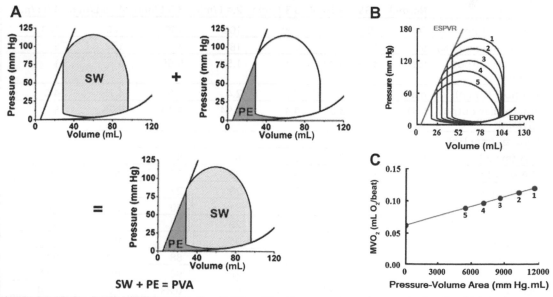

Fig. 2. (*A*) Myocardial oxygen consumption is proportional to pressure-volume area (PVA), which is the sum of external stroke work (SW) and end-systolic potential energy (PE). At a given contractile state, when PVA is varied by changes in loading condition (as in *B*), there is a linear relationship between PVA and myocardial oxygen consumption (MVO_2) on a per beat basis (as in *panel C*).

settings, it is important to understand how circulatory support strategies impact MAP.

Cardiogenic Shock

In the discussions to follow, the impact of various percutaneous circulatory support strategies will be illustrated and compared in a state of acute CGS with pulmonary edema for which representative PV loops and relations are shown by the red lines in **Fig. 1**. With acute CGS as would occur in the setting of a large myocardial infarction, ventricular contractility is markedly reduced, as represented by the downward shift of the ESPVR. In the acute setting, ventricular diastolic properties are not influenced significantly, so the EDPVR would be unchanged. The immediate effects of reduced contractility are decreased blood pressure (manifest as decreased height of the PV loop) and decreased stroke volume (decreased width of the PV loop). With activation of baroreflexes, there are increases in heart rate (with a decrease in the duration of the cardiac cycle, T) increases in TPR, and venoconstriction leading to a marked increases in left ventricular EDP and EDV. The increase in HR (ie, decrease in T) and

decrease in TPR result in a significant increase in Ea. All of these changes are readily identified in **Fig. 1** by the PV loop and ESPVR in red. The resulting hemodynamic parameters for this example derived from the simulation in comparison to the normal condition are summarized in **Table 1**. Consistent with a state of CGS, systolic arterial pressure, cardiac output (CO), and thus CPO and PVA are all decreased and pulmonary capillary pressure is markedly increased.

HEMODYNAMIC EFFECTS OF DIFFERENT PERCUTANEOUS SUPPORT STRATEGIES

The PV framework reviewed above is particularly useful for demonstrating and comparing the hemodynamic effects and metabolic consequences of different percutaneous support devices. The hemodynamic and metabolic impact of a support device depends on the flow rate of the pump and whether blood is pumped from the left ventricle (LV), the left atrium (LA), or the right atrium (RA).The effects of pumping can also depend on the hemodynamic state from which support is initiated, which can vary from near normal (in the case of prophylactic use) to a state of deep CGS.

Table 1
Hemodynamic parameters derived from a cardiovascular model simulating normal conditions, CGS, and then CGS with the addition of different types of circulatory support devices

Hemodynamic Parameter	Normal	CGS	+IABP	LA → Ao 3.3 L/min	LV → Ao 2.4 L/min	LV → Ao 3.5 L/min	LV → Ao 4.75 L/min	RA → Ao 4.0 L/min
Heart rate (bpm)	70	100	100	100	100	100	100	100
Ejection fraction (%)	55	20	22	6	18	17	18	5
LV cardiac output (L/min)	5.31	3.49	3.89	1.14	1.57	0.65	0	1
VAD flow (L/min)	n/a	n/a	n/a	3.3	2.4	3.5	4.75	4.0
Total cardiac output (L/min)	5.31	3.49	3.89	4.4	3.94	4.19	4.74	5
Pressures (mm Hg)								
RA (mean)	8	8	8	9	8	8	9	5
PA systolic	27	39	38	37	38	37	36	40
PA diastolic	13	30	29	26	28	27	25	36
PA mean	16	32	31	29	31	30	28	37
PCP	13	30	29	26	28	27	25	36
Ao systolic	110	92	88	102	95	96	102	110
Ao diastolic	58	67	97	91	81	88	101	99
Ao mean	78	77	86	95	86	90	101	103
CPO (Watts)	0.92	0.60	0.74	0.94	0.76	0.83	1.07	1.14
PVA (mm Hg, mL)	10,363	7850	7637	7878	7537	7290	6860	8700

Abbreviations: Ao, aorta; IABP, intraaortic balloon pump; PA, pulmonary artery; PCP, pulmonary capillary pressure; VAD, ventricular assist device.

Although the first-line therapy for all forms of he-modynamic compromise usually involves medical management with inotropic agents and/or pres-sors,[19,20] these are not discussed here because the focus of this article is on hemodynamic effects of circulatory assist devices, not on the treatment of CGS per se. Nevertheless, it is noteworthy that although shown to increase blood pressure and cardiac output, the impact of such medical therapies on end-organ perfusion can be variable (depending on the degree of peripheral vasocon-striction) and they have well-established adverse effects on the heart itself.[1–5,21,22] Indeed, the com-bination of multiple agents seems to be associated with worse outcome.[22] The effects of intravenous inotropes within the PV framework have been dis-cussed previously.[7]

This review focuses on the currently available forms of percutaneous circulatory support, in-cluding counterpulsation, extracorporeal circula-tory support, and intracorporeal transaortic valvular circulatory support.

Counterpulsation

Counterpulsation with intra-aortic balloon pump-ing is often used in patients with otherwise untreat-able myocardial ischemia (eg, unstable angina) and also in patients with hemodynamic compro-mise as an adjunct to medical therapy (pressors and/or inotropes). A balloon with inflation volume of up to ∼40 mL alternately inflates during diastole and deflates during systole (**Fig. 3**A). Systolic balloon deflation is intended to reduce the pres-sure (and therefore the effective afterload) against which the heart ejects to improve cardiac output. Diastolic balloon inflation is intended to increase aortic pressure to increase coronary blood flow

and end-organ perfusion. The theoretical effects of counterpulsation on the PV loop and hemody-namics are summarized in **Fig. 3**B and **Table 1**. As seen, the effects on parameters like cardiac output (∼10%) and pulmonary capillary pressure (∼1 mm Hg) are small (and may be beyond the sensitivity of detection in the clinical setting), whereas the effects of counterpulsation on coro-nary pressure, and therefore coronary flow, can be significant. Consistent with the conclusions, re-sults of several clinical studies have confirmed no significant hemodynamic effectiveness of counter-pulsation in CGS.[23–26] From an energetic stand-point, there is also a small (∼3%) reduction in PVA, implying that counterpulsation would not significantly reduce myocardial oxygen demands. Nevertheless, there can be a significant increase in CPO owing to the increase in blood pressure. Despite this, however the results of a recent large randomized study showed no survival benefit from counterpulsation in CGS.[27]

Extracorporeal LA-to-Arterial Circulatory Support

Percutaneous LA-to-arterial circulatory support devices (eg, as with the TandemHeart device [CardiacAssist, Pittsburgh, PA, USA]) have signifi-cant beneficial effects on hemodynamic parame-ters, as illustrated in **Fig. 4** and **Table 1** and shown in prior clinical studies.[28,29] Such devices have flow capacities approaching 4 L/min and because they draw blood directly from the LA, pul-monary capillary pressure is reduced significantly, by 4 mm Hg in the present example. Accordingly, LV EDV and pressure are also decreased because blood is diverted from flowing through the mitral valve. At the same time, there is now a continuous

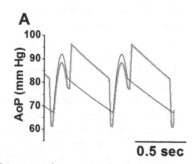
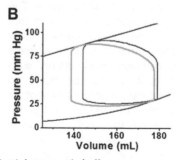

Fig. 3. Theoretical impact of counterpulsation with a 40 mL intra-aortic balloon pump on arterial pressure (*A*) and PV loop (*B*) in CGS. Baseline CGS hemodynamic state described in **Fig. 1** (shown in *red*) isused as a starting point to assess the effects of different circulatory support strategies. During counterpulsation (shown in *green*) balloon deflation decreases blood pressure during ejection (reduced effective ventricular afterload) and balloon inflation during diastole increases arterial pressure with the goal of improving coronary and end-organ perfu-sion. The impact of counterperfusion on the PV loop (panel *B*) shows the reduction in peak ventricular pressure and relatively small effect on stroke volume and EDV. Refer to **Table 1** for more detailed summary of hemody-namic effects.

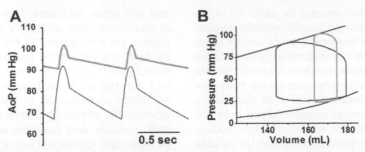

Fig. 4. Impact of left atrial-to-arterial circulatory support strategy on arterial pressure (*A*) and PV loop (*B*). This approach creates a significant increase in diastolic more than systolic arterial pressure (with reduction in PP). There is a significant reduction in LV EDV and pressure. PVA, however, is not significantly altered because of the offsetting effects of the increase in afterload and reduction in preload. Refer to **Table 1** for more detailed summary of hemodynamic effects.

flow of blood to the aorta throughout the cardiac cycle, even during diastole, which has the effect of increasing aortic diastolic pressure and decreasing aortic pulse pressure (PP, which is systolic minus diastolic pressure; **Fig. 4**A). As a consequence of the decrease in LV preload and increase in LV afterload, intrinsic cardiac output from the LV is decreased substantially. Thus, although cardiac output was 3.5 L/min before initiation of support and the extracorporeal system is pumping 3.3 L/min, the final total output during support is not 3.5 + 3.3 = 6.8 L/min, but is 4.4 L/min, an increase of only 1.1 L/min because intrinsic output from the LV decreased from 3.5 to 1.1 L/min due to the effects of the assist device. The reduction of cardiac output is reflected as a decrease in stroke volume (the width of the PV loop) and, accordingly, a reduction in ejection fraction (EF). This example therefore illustrates 2 important and fundamental principles of circulatory support:

1. The final total cardiac output achieved after implantation of partial support circulatory assist device is not the sum of the original cardiac output plus the flow of the assist device. The final cardiac output depends on many factors and, as discussed previously, no general statement can be made as to the expected increase in CO following initiation of circulatory support.[30] In addition, it should specifically be noted that the total cardiac output cannot be determined through examination of the PV loop. Naturally, when the assist device is powerful enough to overtake and pump more than the native heart, the assist device alone determines the total flow.
2. When such a device is used, the marked changes in preload and afterload that result in reductions in intrinsic stroke volume and cardiac output can result in a decrease in EF. Such a reduction does not reflect a reduction in ventricular contractility. As shown in **Fig. 4**,

the end-systolic PV point falls on the same ESPVR, indicating the constancy of LV contractility. The change in EF is purely a result of the change in loading conditions induced during circulatory assist.

In addition to the impact on pulmonary capillary pressure, cardiac output, and diastolic blood pressure, the increase in total cardiac output also results in an overall increase in blood pressure throughout the cardiac cycle, which has the potential benefits of improving coronary blood flow and end-organ perfusion. This approach also results in a substantial increase in CPO, to normal values in this example. On the other hand, there is little impact on PVA (in particular, no significant reduction), principally because of the significant increase in arterial pressure. Accordingly, it is expected that there is little effect on myocardial oxygen consumption with this strategy.

Extracorporeal RA-to-Arterial Circulatory Support

RA-to-arterial circulatory assist devices are becoming increasingly used for patients with severe hemodynamic compromise as with biventricular failure and with pulmonary dysfunction, typically in combination with membrane oxygenation and sometimes with a heat exchanger. Specialized catheters for venous and arterial access are readily available for this application (venous-to-venous pumping configurations, used in patients in whom oxygenation or hypercapnea is the primary problem instead of hemodynamic compromise, is not discussed in this article). Regardless of configuration, these systems are generically referred to as extracorporeal membrane oxygenation systems. The pumps typically used in these circuits are powerful and capable of overtaking the native heart, but are generally set at ~4 L/min. There are distinct hemodynamic differences between sourcing the blood from the RA as opposed to the LA that was discussed in the prior section. The major difference, readily appreciated from the PV loop (**Fig. 5**, see **Table 1**), is that when applied to patients with compromised LV function, this configuration can result in further significant and potentially detrimental increases in pulmonary capillary and left ventricular end-diastolic pressures and LV distension can result. Because of this, some form of LV venting may be required, although not generally able to be implemented percutaneously (see further discussion of this later). This LV loading effects is because with RA-to-arterial circulatory support the only path for blood to leave the LV is via the aortic valve and to overcome the significantly elevated arterial pressure in the setting of the decreased contractility, that can only occur at high (higher than starting) levels of ventricular preload. Accordingly, whereas with LA-to-arterial pumping the higher the flow rate, the greater the degree of ventricular unloading, with RA-to-arterial pumping, the higher the flow rate, the greater the degree of ventricular loading. These increases in preload result in further increases in PVA and, therefore, in oxygen consumption. Confirmation of this loading effect of extracorporeal membrane oxygenation was recently reported by Kawashima and coworkers, who noted consistent elevation of PVA in an animal model of varying degrees of LV failure.[26]

Intracorporeal Transaortic Valve Circulatory Support

The final class of percutaneous circulatory support devices to be considered is the pumps placed at the ends of catheters that source blood from the LV and pump it to the aorta. Although the Hemopump was the first device developed specifically with this mode of action, technical problems prevented that particular device from being a viable

clinical product.[31] More recently, the Impella (Abiomed, Danvers, MA, USA) class of devices has been introduced and is now being used on a routine basis.[32] Three different sized pumps are available, each with its own maximum pumping capacity: 2.5, 4.0, and 5.0 L/min. Because all 3 devices use an LV-to-aorta support strategy, the impact on hemodynamics and myocardial energetics are fundamentally the same, becoming more "potent" in both respects as the flow rate is increased.

The impact of LV-to-aorta pumping on the PV loop, illustrated in **Fig. 6**B (with pumping rates of 2.4 L/min in green, 3.5 L/min in orange, and 4.75 L/min in magenta), is fundamentally different than the other support strategies. Specifically, because these devices are pumping blood continuously out of the LV into the aorta independent of the phase of the cardiac cycle, there are no isovolumic contraction or isovolumic relaxation periods; the loop transforms from a more or less rectangular shape to a triangular shape, especially at the highest pumping rates. Also, as pumping speed is increased, there is a progressively greater leftward shift of the loop to lower ventricular EDVs and EDPs, corresponding with progressively smaller PVAs and, therefore, progressively lower levels of myocardial oxygen demand.

As with the other support systems, the impact on CO cannot be determined from the PV loop because both the heart and the device contribute to the total flow to the body. As summarized in **Table 1**, native CO flow decreases as pump flow increases but total flow and MAP increase, which has the potential to improve coronary[33] and end-organ perfusion. With the device pumping 2.4 L/min, native CO decreases by ~1/3 but total output increases by ~0.5 L/min and there is an ~10 mm Hg increase in MAP. As shown in **Fig. 6**A, the increase in MAP is due almost entirely to an increase in diastolic pressure with very little increase in systolic pressure; accordingly, PP decreases. The rise in diastolic pressure is due to

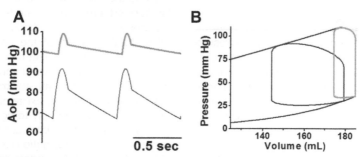

Fig. 5. Impact of right atrial-to-arterial circulatory support strategy on arterial pressure (*A*) and PV loop (*B*). This approach creates a significant increase in diastolic more than systolic arterial pressure (with reduction in PP). There is a significant increase in LV EDV and pressure. Consequently, there is ventricular overloading and PVA increases. Refer to **Table 1** for more detailed summary of hemodynamic effects.

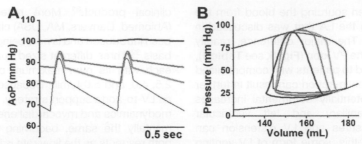

Fig. 6. Impact of left ventricular-to-arterial circulatory support strategy on arterial pressure (*A*) and PV loop (*B*). Three levels of support are shown: 2.4 L/min (*green*), 3.5 L/min (*orange*), and 4.75 L/min (*magenta*). This approach creates a significant increase in diastolic pressure with little impact on systolic arterial pressure until the degree of support is sufficient to overtake the natural heart. There is a significant reduction in LV EDV and pressure that increases as the magnitude of support increases. Note that the PV loop loses its normal rectangular shape in favor of an increasingly triangular shape as the magnitude of support increases. PVA decreases in relation to the amount of flow from the device. Refer to **Table 1** for more detailed summary of hemodynamic effects.

continual pumping of blood from the LV to aorta during diastole.

With pump flow increased to 3.5 L/min and the further reduction in EDV and EDP, total flow is increased by 0.7 L/min above the starting CGS value as native CO decreases to only 0.65 L/min. MAP increases further, again due to further increased diastolic pressure with a relatively small increase in systolic pressure and a further reduction in PP.

Finally, with the device pumping 4.75 L/min, the native heart is overcome and all of the flow is from the pump. The LV cannot generate pressure to overcome arterial pressure and the aortic valve stays closed. Accordingly, the arterial pressure loses pulsatility, with only minimal fluctuations from slight variations in pump output caused by time-dependent changes in LV-to-aorta pressure gradients during the cardiac cycle. It is appreciated on the PV diagram that despite the fact that the heart is not ejecting into the aorta, there are still cycle-dependent changes in ventricular volume owing to pressure-dependent opening and closing of the mitral valve in response to ventricular contraction and pressure variations.

Other Considerations

The discussions above have been based on results obtained from a cardiovascular simulation.[8,30] Although validated to a certain extent, the behavior of the real cardiovascular system is significantly more complex than can be captured in any such simulation. Furthermore, there is significant variability in hemodynamic characteristics from patient to patient. Even then, the predicted effects do not account for changes in patient status following initiation of circulatory support that can be mediated by baroreflexes, changes in renal function, the multitude of drugs that are used in

different clinical scenarios, and many other factors. The presence of valvular lesions, not considered at all, can have a profound effect on device performance. Finally, only one particular hemodynamic profile of CGS has been considered; there are infinite possible combinations of ventricular and vascular dysfunction with which patients present. As emphasized at the start, the impact of any circulatory support system is highly dependent on native cardiovascular properties. As just one example, the impact of circulatory support in CGS in the absence of profound elevations in pulmonary capillary pressure is quantitatively very different with regard to changes in ventricular EDV and EDP achieved with the different support strategies.

The hemodynamic demands surrounding the prophylactic use of temporary percutaneous support are significantly more modest than those related to their use in CGS, both in terms of hemodynamic and duration of use requirements. These hemodynamic demands have been discussed previously[34] and have not been reviewed here.

Finally, although the fundamental principles underlying the use of such devices for right ventricular support are similar, there are many unique features of such applications, especially as they relate to the nature of the underlying hemodynamic abnormalities being treated. These factors, in combination with several important differences between right and left ventricular physiology, caution against simple extrapolation of concepts discussed above to apply to right-sided support.

Taking all of this into account, one should consider that the information reviewed above provides a framework for understanding basic hemodynamic concepts of circulatory support and not that it provides generally applicable quantitative information about the hemodynamic effects of any particular circulatory support device in any particular patient. To take this approach to that level, one potentially fruitful line of investigation is to develop such computer simulations further to be able to model specific patients and be able to predict the hemodynamic effects of specific interventions (ie, development of algorithms for pathophysiology-based personalized medicine). Initial work on such an approach has already been started[30] but requires significant further development and validation.

SUMMARY

Four different approaches to circulatory support have been reviewed. Each approach has a distinct hemodynamic fingerprint with regard to effects on the ventricular PV loop, cardiac output, arterial pressure, pulmonary capillary pressure, PVA, and myocardial oxygen consumption. An understanding of basic hemodynamic concepts and mechanisms that lead to hemodynamic compromise (including hypotension, hypoperfusion, and elevated venous pressures) provides a foundation for understanding how different modes of circulatory support impact key cardiovascular parameters in various clinical settings. Such understanding can help guide the choice of which device is most appropriate for a given patient.

This is particularly important because in percutaneous circulatory support there are very few randomized clinical trials to guide therapeutic decisions. With the lack of such evidence to establish treatment guidelines, therapeutic decision-making is based on first principles and, ultimately, experience.

Consistent with prior clinical trials,[29,35] the hemodynamic effects of counterpulsation seem to be mainly restricted to effects on blood pressure. Whether this results in any clinical secondary benefits beyond reducing myocardial ischemia is unknown.[27]

Most active percutaneous circulatory support systems provide partial support in that they do not completely take over heart function. Rather, these devices generally work in concert with the native heart. When operating in this mode, the final total CO is not the sum of the cardiac output before initiation of support plus the flow of the device. The resulting changes in LV preload and afterload generally reduce intrinsic CO and the final total CO is determined by the complex interactions between heart, vasculature, and device.

When the device overtakes the intrinsic pumping capacity of the heart, the aortic valve remains closed and CO is determined exclusively by the heart.

With an LA-to-arterial support strategy, the greater the amount of pumping, the greater the increase in MAP and the greater the reduction in ventricular preload. With an RA-to-arterial strategy, the greater the amount of pumping, the greater the increase in MAP but the greater the potential for increasing ventricular preload. With an LV-to-aorta strategy, the more you pump, the more you reduce both ventricular preload and MAP; minimization of increases in systolic arterial pressure with this approach in comparison to the LA-to-arterial pumping strategy seems to make this approach more effective in reducing PVA and, potentially, myocardial oxygen consumption.

Although some of these conclusions may seem trivial, it is an understanding of the underlying theories that have the potential to guide future researchers in optimization of therapies, help generate hypotheses for clinical trials, and help guide choice of the proper device for specific clinical trials that will ultimately provide evidence required to guide therapeutic decision-making.

REFERENCES

1. Cuffe MS, Califf RM, Adams KF Jr, et al. Short-term intravenous milrinone for acute exacerbation of chronic heart failure: a randomized controlled trial. JAMA 2002;287:1541–7.
2. Abraham WT, Adams KF, Fonarow GC, et al. In-hospital mortality in patients with acute decompensated heart failure requiring intravenous vasoactive medications: an analysis from the Acute Decompensated Heart Failure National Registry (ADHERE). J Am Coll Cardiol 2005;46:57–64.
3. Dunser MW, Hasibeder WR. Sympathetic overstimulation during critical illness: adverse effects of adrenergic stress. J Intensive Care Med 2009;24:293–316.
4. Goldspink DF, Burniston JG, Ellison GM, et al. Catecholamine-induced apoptosis and necrosis in cardiac and skeletal myocytes of the rat in vivo: the same or separate death pathways? Exp Physiol 2004;89:407–16.
5. Culling W, Penny WJ, Cunliffe G, et al. Arrhythmogenic and electrophysiological effects of alpha adrenoceptor stimulation during myocardial ischaemia and reperfusion. J Mol Cell Cardiol 1987;19:251–8.
6. Burkhoff D, Mirsky I, Suga H. Assessment of systolic and diastolic ventricular properties via pressure-volume analysis: a guide for clinical, translational, and basic researchers. Am J Physiol Heart Circ Physiol 2005;289:H501–12.
7. Burkhoff D, Naidu SS. The science behind percutaneous hemodynamic support: a review and comparison of support strategies. Catheter Cardiovasc Interv 2012;80:816–29.

8. Burkhoff D, Tyberg JV. Why does pulmonary venous pressure rise following the onset of left ventricular dysfunction: a theoretical analysis. Am J Physiol 1993;265(HCP 34):H1819–28.

9. Sunagawa K, Maughan WL, Burkhoff D, et al. Left ventricular interaction with arterial load studied in isolated canine ventricle. Am J Physiol 1983; 245(HCP 14):H773–80.

10. Fincke R, Hochman JS, Lowe AM, et al. Cardiac power is the strongest hemodynamic correlate of mortality in cardiogenic shock: a report from the SHOCK trial registry. J Am Coll Cardiol 2004;44: 340–8.

11. Torgersen C, Schmittinger CA, Wagner S, et al. Hemodynamic variables and mortality in cardiogenic shock: a retrospective cohort study. Crit Care 2009;13:R157.

12. Mendoza DD, Cooper HA, Panza JA. Cardiac power output predicts mortality across a broad spectrum of patients with acute cardiac disease. Am Heart J 2007;153:366–70.

13. Chatterjee K. Coronary hemodynamics in heart failure and effects of therapeutic interventions. J Card Fail 2009;15:116–23.

14. Suga H. Total mechanical energy of a ventricle model and cardiac oxygen consumption. Am J Physiol 1979;236:H498–505.

15. Takaoka H, Takeuchi M, Odake M, et al. Comparison of hemodynamic determinants for myocardial oxygen consumption under different contractile states in human ventricle. Circulation 1993;87:59–69.

16. Schipke JD, Burkhoff D, Kass DA, et al. Hemodynamic dependence of myocardial oxygen consumption indices. Am J Physiol 1990;258(HCP 27): H1281–91.

17. Krams R, Sipkema P, Zegers J, et al. Contractility is the main determinant of coronary systolic flow impediment. Am J Physiol 1989;257:H1936–44.

18. Krams R, Sipkema P, Westerhof N. Varying elastance concept may explain coronary systolic flow impediment. Am J Physiol 1989;257:H1471–9.

19. Petersen JW, Felker GM. Inotropes in the management of acute heart failure. Crit Care Med 2008;36: S106–11.

20. El Mokhtari NE, Arlt A, Meissner A, et al. Inotropic therapy for cardiac low output syndrome: comparison of hemodynamic effects of dopamine/dobutamine versus dopamine/dopexamine. Eur J Med Res 2008;13:459–63.

21. de Backer D, Biston P, Devriendt J, et al. Comparison of dopamine and norepinephrine in the treatment of shock. N Engl J Med 2010;362:779–89.

22. Samuels LE, Kaufman MS, Thomas MP, et al. Pharmacological criteria for ventricular assist device insertion following postcardiotomy shock: experience with the Abiomed BVS system. J Card Surg 1999;14:288–93.

23. Sauren LD, Accord RE, Hamzeh K, et al. Combined Impella and intra-aortic balloon pump support to improve both ventricular unloading and coronary blood flow for myocardial recovery: an experimental study. Artif Organs 2007;31:839–42.

24. Reesink KD, Dekker AL, Van Ommen V, et al. Miniature intracardiac assist device provides more effective cardiac unloading and circulatory support during severe left heart failure than intraaortic balloon pumping. Chest 2004;126:896–902.

25. Seyfarth M, Sibbing D, Bauer I, et al. A randomized clinical trial to evaluate the safety and efficacy of a percutaneous left ventricular assist device versus intra-aortic balloon pumping for treatment of cardiogenic shock caused by myocardial infarction. J Am Coll Cardiol 2008;52:1584–8.

26. Kawashima D, Gojo S, Nishimura T, et al. Left ventricular mechanical support with Impella provides more ventricular unloading in heart failure than extracorporeal membrane oxygenation. ASAIO J 2011;57:169–76.

27. Thiele H, Zeymer U, Neumann FJ, et al. Intraaortic balloon support for myocardial infarction with cardiogenic shock. N Engl J Med 2012;367:1287–96.

28. Burkhoff D, O'Neill W, Brunckhorst C, et al. Feasibility study of the use of the TandemHeart percutaneous ventricular assist device for treatment of cardiogenic shock. Catheter Cardiovasc Interv 2006;68:211–7.

29. Burkhoff D, Cohen H, Brunckhorst C, et al. A randomized multicenter clinical study to evaluate the safety and efficacy of the TandemHeart percutaneous ventricular assist device versus conventional therapy with intraaortic balloon pumping for treatment of cardiogenic shock. Am Heart J 2006;152:469.e1–8.

30. Morley D, Litwak K, Ferber P, et al. Hemodynamic effects of partial ventricular support in chronic heart failure: results of simulation validated with in vivo data. J Thorac Cardiovasc Surg 2007;133:21–8.

31. Sweeney MS. The Hemopump in 1997: a clinical, political, and marketing evolution. Ann Thorac Surg 1999;68:761–3.

32. Raess DH, Weber DM. Impella 2.5. J Cardiovasc Transl Res 2009;2:168–72.

33. Remmelink M, Sjauw KD, Henriques JP, et al. Effects of left ventricular unloading by Impella recover LP2.5 on coronary hemodynamics. Catheter Cardiovasc Interv 2007;70:532–7.

34. O'Neill WW, Kleiman NS, Moses J, et al. A prospective, randomized clinical trial of hemodynamic support with Impella 2.5 versus intra-aortic balloon pump in patients undergoing high-risk percutaneous coronary intervention: the PROTECT II study. Circulation 2012;126:1717–27.

35. Thiele H, Lauer B, Hambrecht R, et al. Reversal of cardiogenic shock by percutaneous left atrial-to-femoral arterial bypass assistance. Circulation 2001;104:2917–22.

Usage of Percutaneous Left Ventricular Assist Devices in Clinical Practice and High-risk Percutaneous Coronary Intervention

Juan N. Pulido, MD[a,b], Charanjit S. Rihal, MD[c],*

KEYWORDS

- Percutaneous left ventricular assist devices • Coronary interventions • Shock • High risk

KEY POINTS

- High-risk patients with complex coronary anatomy and depressed left ventricular function benefit most from surgical revascularization.
- The highest risk patients are frequently deemed inoperable and have limited therapeutic options.
- Prophylactic use of intra-aortic balloon pumps (IABPs) is the most common and traditionally the preferred method of circulatory assistance for high-risk percutaneous coronary interventions. However, they provide limited hemodynamic support.
- Percutaneous left ventricular assist devices (pLVADs) such as the TandemHeart and the Impella provide superior hemodynamic support compared with IABPs.
- Unique hemodynamic benefits from pLVADs include maintenance of cardiac output, active left ventricular (LV) unloading with reduction of LV filling pressures, and, crucially, preservation of vital organ perfusion.

INTRODUCTION

Coronary artery bypass grafting (CABG) is usually the therapy of choice for revascularization in patients with severe left ventricular (LV) systolic dysfunction or complex coronary lesions, including multivessel disease and left main or equivalent disease.[1] However, many of these patients are at high surgical risk and surgery may be declined because of unacceptable risks of morbidity and mortality. This patient population is left with limited options because cardiovascular complications during percutaneous revascularization are high as well. This risk is largely caused by the imminent hemodynamic collapse that can occur during balloon inflations, stent deployment, or rotational atherectomy. Coronary artery dissection with vessel occlusion or no reflow may quickly result in patient demise.

Although there is no current unifying definition of the term high-risk percutaneous coronary intervention (HR-PCI), it is well recognized that patients with 1 or more of the following characteristics qualify as high risk: (1) severe LV systolic dysfunction, (2) multivessel disease and left main or equivalent coronary artery disease, (3) heavily calcified coronary arteries, and (4) previous CABG with severe graft disease. Emergent procedures for

[a] Division of Cardiovascular Anesthesia, Department of Anesthesiology, Mayo Clinic, 200 1st Street Southwest, Rochester, MN 55905, USA; [b] Division of Critical Care Medicine, Department of Anesthesiology, Mayo Clinic, 200 1st Street Southwest, Rochester, MN 55905, USA; [c] Division of Cardiovascular Diseases, Department of Medicine, Mayo Clinic, 200 1st Street Southwest, Rochester, MN 55905, USA
* Corresponding author.
E-mail address: rihal@mayo.edu

Intervent Cardiol Clin 2 (2013) 417–428
http://dx.doi.org/10.1016/j.iccl.2013.04.002
2211-7458/13/$ – see front matter © 2013 Elsevier Inc. All rights reserved.

ongoing myocardial ischemia are also associated with an increased risk of adverse events with PCI. As such, patients with post–myocardial infarction (MI) cardiogenic shock, represent the highest risk patient population (**Box 1**).

This article discusses the principles and rationale for percutaneous LV assist devices (pLVADs). The different devices are described, including the intra-aortic balloon pump (IABP), available pLVADs, portable extracorporeal membrane oxygenation (ECMO) support, and their role in the management of patients undergoing HR-PCI.

RATIONALE AND INDICATIONS FOR PLVADS

The mechanism by which pLVADs provide unique ventricular support is primarily based on reduction of LV stroke work by actively unloading the LV while maintaining systemic and coronary perfusion (**Fig. 1**). These effects translate into a favorable balance of myocardial supply and demand. Benefits from these devices have been reported in patients undergoing pLVAD-supported HR-PCI.[2–5] Although the currently available devices provide different mechanisms of LV support, pLVADs have the following beneficial effects to a varying degree depending on the device used:

1. Reduction of LV stroke work
2. LV pressure and volume unloading with enhanced remodeling capability
3. Decreased wall tension with improved endocardial blood flow
4. Reduced metabolic requirements from unloaded beating heart
5. Preservation of peripheral organ and skeletal muscle perfusion
6. Presumed enhanced ability for cellular repair and survival

The IABP is the traditional method of choice for mechanical circulatory assistance in patients in cardiogenic shock following MI[6] or patients undergoing HR-PCI.[7] By displacing blood in the descending aorta during inflation in diastole, the IABP increases coronary perfusion, which is followed by a vacuum effect during deflation facilitating LV ejection, resulting in reduced LV afterload and increased stroke volume. Minimal or no reduction in LV stroke work occurs (see **Fig. 1**). This device is limited by the lack of active cardiac support and the need for accurate synchronization with the cardiac cycle.

In addition, although ECMO provides partial to full cardiopulmonary support, it is rarely used in HR-PCI unless emergent need caused by imminent or present cardiopulmonary failure. However, there is a lack of active LV unloading and ECMO may increase afterload because of retrograde aortic flow without left atrial decompression. The hemodynamic effects of these devices are summarized in **Table 1**.

The therapeutic goal when instituting mechanical circulatory support is to restore or maintain hemodynamics and systemic perfusion during HR-PCI or in patients with cardiogenic shock with severe cardiac failure (see **Table 1**).

PERCUTANEOUS CIRCULATORY SUPPORT
Intra-aortic Balloon Pump

Since the introduction of a percutaneous IABP in 1980,[8] intra-aortic balloon counterpulsation has become the most frequently used mechanical circulatory assist device in the world.[9] LV systolic unloading and diastolic augmentation with resultant improvements in coronary flow are the generally accepted mechanisms of action. IABP counterpulsation is the classic mechanical support device used for HR-PCI and is also used in a variety of surgical and nonsurgical patients with cardiogenic shock, either as a perioperative circulatory assist device, or in the setting of acute coronary syndrome.

Indications
Current indications for IABP include hemodynamic support for cardiogenic shock, refractory unstable angina, stabilization of left main coronary artery disease, mechanical complications of acute MI, HR-PCI, and preoperative stabilization for high-risk cardiac surgery.[7,10]

Implantation and device description
The IABP is a double-lumen 7.5-French to 8.0-French catheter with a 25-mL to 50-mL polyethylene balloon at the distal end and a pump console to drive the balloon inflation. It is inserted percutaneously via the femoral artery and advanced to 2 to 3 cm distal to the origin of the left subclavian artery. Final position is confirmed with fluoroscopy. The inner lumen is used to monitor arterial pressure and the outer lumen is used for gas delivery

---

Box 1
Determinants of HR-PCI

1. Severe LV systolic dysfunction
2. Multivessel disease and left main or equivalent coronary artery disease
3. Heavily calcified coronary arteries
4. Previous CABG with severe graft disease
5. Ongoing myocardial ischemia
6. Post-MI cardiogenic shock

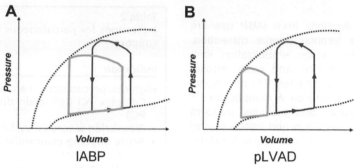

Fig. 1. LV pressure-volume loop comparing effects of IABP versus pLVAD support. Pressure-volume loop representing 1 cardiac cycle. Red, steady state; blue, with mechanical support. (*A*) IABP. Note that stroke volume is augmented and stroke work is not reduced. (*B*) pLVAD. Note the active unloading by reduction of stroke volume, stroke work, and filling pressures.

from the console. Helium is the most commonly used gas because of its low density and favorable physical properties. Complete balloon expansion should be confirmed on initiation of counterpulsation with fluoroscopy and peripheral pulses should be assessed to ensure adequate limb perfusion.

The balloon should inflate after aortic valve closure (corresponding with the dicrotic notch on the arterial pressure waveform) and deflate immediately before aortic valve opening (corresponding with the nadir before the systolic upstroke). The

frequency of balloon counterpulsation can be timed to augment every beat (1:1) to every third beat (1:3).

Contraindications

The IABP is contraindicated in patients with significant aortic regurgitation or aortic dissection. Relative contraindications for femoral percutaneous insertion include the presence of severe peripheral arterial disease, coagulopathy, abdominal or thoracoabdominal aortic aneurysms, and the presence of femoral-popliteal bypass grafts.

Table 1
Hemodynamic effects of percutaneous mechanical circulatory support devices

Device	Type of Circulatory Support	Hemodynamic Effects
IABP	Balloon counterpulsation Diastolic inflation	Increased coronary blood flow Decreased myocardial oxygen demand Decreased myocardial wall stress Increased cardiac output
TandemHeart	In-parallel circulatory support • LA: femoral arterial bypass	Active circulatory support Active increase in cardiac output Active LV unloading Decreased LV stroke work Decreased myocardial oxygen demand Decreased myocardial wall stress
Impella	In-parallel circulatory support • Transvalvular (LV: aortic) axial flow pump	Active circulatory support Active increase of cardiac output Active LV unloading Decreased LV stroke work Decreased myocardial oxygen demand Decreased myocardial wall stress
ECMO (venoarterial)	Partial to full cardiopulmonary bypass	Active circulatory support Partial to full cardiopulmonary support Provision of ventilation and oxygenation Lack of active LV unloading caused by retrograde aortic flow May increase LV afterload and myocardial wall stress

Abbreviation: LA, left atrium.

Complications

Most of the complications from IABP use are vascular, including femoral arterial dissection, arteriovenous fistula creation, embolization, limb ischemia, bleeding, infection, and, rarely, stroke. It is estimated that approximately 7% of patients who require IABP experience a complication.[10] Vigilance is mandatory and includes frequent assessment of limb perfusion and infection, and monitoring of coagulation. As with any support device, the incidence of complications increases with the duration of use.

Role of IABP counterpulsation in HR-PCI

The IABP is the most common form of percutaneous of circulatory support in high-risk patients undergoing PCI. Nonetheless, despite the earlier suggestion of reduced mortality and complication rate in elective IABP use during HR-PCI by observational studies,[11] a larger multicenter prospective randomized trial has failed to confirm this early hypothesis for patients undergoing HR-PCI[12]; despite having a class I indication for use in patients with post-MI cardiogenic shock, its used has been also challenged recently in the IABP-SHOCK[13] and IABP-SHOCK II[14] (Intra-aortic Balloon Counter Pulsation in Myocardial Infarction Related Shock) trials. However, the BCIS-1 (Balloon Pump Assisted Coronary Intervention Study) trial compared elective IABP use for HR-PCI versus provisional use, in which the IABP was available and ready to use in case of hemodynamic instability, and 12% of the control arm required rescue IABP insertion for prolonged hypotension.[12] Although the results of this study do not support routine use of elective IABP for HR-PCI, the high crossover rate in the provisional arm suggests that the interventional team should be prepared for emergency insertion.

pLVADs

Currently available pLVADs include the Tandem-Heart (Cardiac Assist Technologies, Inc., Pittsburg, PA) and the Impella Circulatory Support System (Abiomed, Danvers, MA). Both devices unload the LV by different mechanisms and have varying degrees of circulatory support depending on the diameter of the cannulas used. Hemodynamic effects and indications are summarized in **Tables 1** and **2**.

The TandemHeart

The TandemHeart (Cardiac Assist Technologies, Inc., Pittsburgh, PA) is a transseptal left atrial to femoral arterial pLVAD that provides in-parallel circulatory support by draining fully oxygenated blood from the left atrium (provided normal lung function) and pumping it retrogradely via the

Table 2
Indications for percutaneous ventricular support
Indication
High-risk percutaneous cardiac procedures   • Complex PCI (left main disease, multivessel PCI)   • Preexisting severe LV dysfunction   • Acute ongoing myocardial ischemia   • Complex radiofrequency ablation procedures for ventricular arrhythmias
Cardiogenic shock   • After MI   • After cardiac surgery   • Chronic heart failure with acute hemodynamic decompensation   • Acute myocarditis   • Myocardial contusion   • Refractory ventricular arrhythmias
Preoperative stabilization for cardiac surgery   • Active myocardial ischemia   • Acute mechanical complications of MI (acute ischemic mitral regurgitation, VSD)   • Severe preoperative LV dysfunction
Bridge to recovery   • After MI   • Post–cardiac surgery myocardial stunning
Bridge to permanent therapy   • Surgically implanted long term LVAD   • Heart transplant

Abbreviations: LVAD, LV assist device; PCI, percutaneous coronary intervention; VSD, ventricular septal defect.

Modified from Pulido JN, Park SJ, Rihal CS. Percutaneous left ventricular assist devices: clinical uses, future applications, and anesthetic considerations. J Cardiovasc Anesth 2010;24(3):478–86; with permission.

femoral artery, reducing cardiac work load, oxygen demand, and LV filling pressure (**Fig. 2**).[15,16] This technique was first described by Dennis[17] in 1962 with venous access from the jugular vein. However, it was not until the 1990s when the transfemoral percutaneous approach of this type of circulatory support for patients undergoing HR-PCI was described for short-term use.[18]

The TandemHeart is a low-speed centrifugal continuous-flow pump that has been approved by the US Food and Drug Administration (FDA) for short-term (6 hours) circulatory support for cardiogenic shock[15,16] and HR-PCI[3,7] and has received CE (European Community) mark for up to 30 days. The percutaneous system is capable of delivering up to 5 L/min of flow at 7500 rpm.

Implantation and device description The Tandem-Heart requires a transseptal puncture with the Brockenbrough needle into the left atrium (LA) via femoral vein access (see **Fig. 2**). The inflow

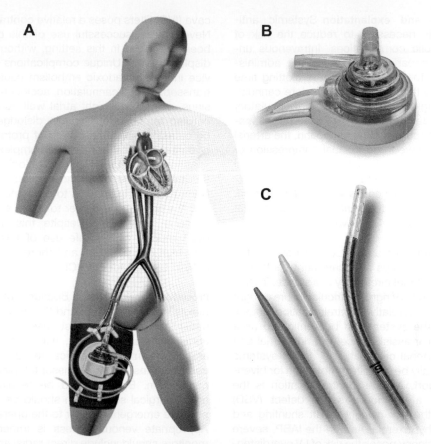

Fig. 2. The TandemHeart (Cardiac Assist Technologies Inc., Pittsburgh, PA). (*A*) The percutaneously inserted device in place. Note the femoral venous transseptal and arterial cannula connected to the TandemHeart centrifugal pump. (*B*) The centrifugal pump. (*C*) The TandemHeart cannulas. (*Courtesy of* CardiacAssist, Pittsburgh, PA; with permission.)

transseptal cannula is a 21-French polyurethane catheter with a large end hole and 14 side holes to facilitate LA decompression. The centrifugal flow pump is a low prime volume device (10 mL) that includes a 6-blade rotating impeller that is powered by a direct-current microprocessor-controlled electromagnetic rotary motor. The system includes 2 controllers, a primary and a backup, which are constantly ready for use and have extensive self-diagnostics with alarm features to ensure continuous support. Built-in batteries allow uninterrupted circulatory assistance for 1 hour to facilitate transport or in case of outage. A pressure transducer is used to monitor the infusion pressure and alerts for potential blockages in the infusion line. The outflow cannula is 15 to 17 French and is inserted in the common femoral artery.

After percutaneous puncture of the femoral vein and standard transseptal puncture and predilation of the fossa ovalis, the venous inflow cannula is inserted in the LA and position is confirmed with contrast injection. Right-to-left shunting can potentially occur if some side holes of the transseptal cannula remain in the right atrium and can be suspected with arterial desaturation. Dislodgement of the atrial cannula can result in sudden systemic desaturation. The arterial inflow cannula is subsequently inserted in the ipsilateral or contralateral common femoral artery using the Seldinger technique and advanced until the tip is in the common iliac artery. Care must be taken to assess arterial caliber with imaging before cannulation. This assessment can be done before the procedure with computed tomography or magnetic resonance, or during the procedure with angiography. After air removal, the cannulas are connected to the centrifugal pump by standard heparin-coated Tygon tubing. Oxygenated blood is retrieved from the LA and pumped into the abdominal aorta via the femoral inflow cannula. The assembly and institution of mechanical circulatory support can be achieved within 30 minutes by experienced operators and usage up to 14 days has been reported.[19,20]

Maintenance and explantation Systemic anti-coagulation is necessary to reduce the risk of thromboembolic complications. Intravenous un-fractionated heparin (100 units/kg) is administered, aiming for an initial activated clotting time (ACT) of more than 300 seconds before cannulation. Following successful weaning of circulatory support, the device can be explanted percutaneously. After discontinuation of heparin, the arterial cannula is removed and manual compression or suture closure of the puncture site is performed until adequate hemostasis is achieved. After explantation of the venous transseptal cannula, there is a small residual atrial septal defect that usually closes within 4 to 6 weeks.[19]

Contraindications As a pure LV assist device, the TandemHeart requires adequate right ventricular function for optimal circulatory assistance. Therefore the presence of right ventricular failure or right ventricular MI is a relative contraindication for use. In contrast, the system can be configured as a right ventricular assist device with right atrial and pulmonary arterial cannulation,[21,22] or 2 systems can theoretically be used in combination for biventricular support. Another contraindication is the presence of a ventricular septal defect (VSD) because of the risk of right-to-left shunting and subsequent hypoxemia. As with the IABP, severe aortic insufficiency poses the risk of LV overdistention and subendocardial ischemia. Like other pLVADs that require percutaneous insertion of large cannulas in the femoral artery, the presence of severe peripheral arterial disease and femoral grafts may preclude the use of this device, as well as any contraindication for systemic anticoagulation. In patients with peripheral vascular disease, the lower extremity may be perfused with a catheter placed antegrade that is perfused via the side port of the main cannula.

Complications and limitations General complications related to the femoral vessel cannulation include bleeding, infection, and limb ischemia.[19] An important limitation is the requirement of large arterial and venous cannulas to achieve adequate circulatory support and the need for transseptal puncture. Transseptal puncture is not performed by all interventional cardiologists, requires a high degree of training and expertise, and is associated with its own set of complications. Nonetheless, there is nothing inherently difficult with transseptal left heart catheterization, and it is being taught in multiple training courses and in academic medical centers with busy structural heart programs.

Moreover, because of the need for femoral venous access, the presence of inferior vena cava (IVC) filters poses a relative contraindication. Nevertheless, successful use of this device has been described in this setting, without IVC filter displacement.[23] Unique complications to this device include paradoxic embolism caused by the transseptal atrial cannulation, accidental coronary sinus, or posterior right atrial wall puncture with cardiac tamponade. Cannula dislodgement can be catastrophic in the setting of profound shock or during a critical portion of a complex PCI.[24]

Although the beneficial physiologic effects of this device have been shown, there have been limited studies in humans to date and none have had the appropriate power to prove a substantial mortality benefit.[25,26] Despite this, there have been reports of the safe use of this device in very-high-risk patients[3] and there is a place for pLVAD support for HR-PCI.[7]

Procedural management Because of the complexity of the procedure and the usual severity of patient comorbidities, most cases are performed under general anesthesia, with adequate preparation for emergent surgical rescue because of complications during transseptal placement or cannulation. Blood should be readily available and a surgical scrub team should be notified for possible emergent transfer to the operating room. Appropriate venous access is imperative, and monitors should include direct radial arterial pressure monitoring, central venous catheter, and pulmonary artery catheter. At first, cardiac output is high with the circulatory support (7–8 L/min) but usually drops during critical portions of the procedure because the LV may stop contracting. In severely compromised patients, the use of transesophageal echocardiography, continuous cardiac output pulmonary artery catheter, or mixed venous oxygen monitor can help tailor the hemodynamic support before, during, and after circulatory support by the pLVAD.

Before insertion of the cannulas, the patient needs to be anticoagulated with a goal of ACT greater than 300 seconds. Unfractionated heparin is usually the anticoagulant of choice; however, direct thrombin inhibitors, such as bivalirudin or argatroban, may be used in cases of contraindication to heparin therapy (heparin-induced thrombocytopenia, and so forth).

Vigilance for complications during cannula placement is vital for effective and timely response. Complications as described earlier, including hypoxemia caused by right-to-left shunt, hypotension, cardiac tamponade, and bleeding can be catastrophic. Before starting the centrifugal pump and adequate deairing, a fluid bolus load of 1 L of isotonic crystalloid solution or 500 mL of colloid is administered to fill the heart at the time of pump start. The low prime volume of the centrifugal pump minimizes the hemodilution effect. Attention for air emboli is crucial because a new atrial septal defect is created.

Inotropic support should be available and ready for use. During emergence, a multidisciplinary approach led by the interventional cardiologist weans the patient from the partial bypass by reducing the revolutions per minute and assisted flow to achieve an approximate mean arterial blood pressure of 70 to 75 mm Hg. At the end of the procedure, the cardiologist removes the cannulas and repairs the vessels, usually with a vascular closure device after reversal of anticoagulation with protamine (if heparin is used).

In patients with atrioventricular conduction abnormalities, consideration should be made to place ventricular pacing wires in case of complete heart block or asystole before circulatory support. If wires are present at the time of cannula insertion, they should be withdrawn before transseptal cannulation or the cardiologist should be notified. In experienced institutions with extensive expertise, the TandemHeart can be readily placed with minimal complications in these cases; consideration to perform the procedure under sedation can be made. However, close communication and constant vigilance by the anesthesia personnel is critical.

Role of the TandemHeart pLVAD in HR-PCI The TandemHeart pLVAD has been successfully used as a bridge to procedure in patients undergoing HR-PCI, in particular in patients with unprotected left main coronary artery and severely depressed LV systolic function.[3,19,27–29] Alli and colleagues[3] described the use of this device in 54 patients undergoing HR-PCI with a 97% procedural success rate and major vascular complications in 13% of patients. In a small, prospective, single-center, randomized trial comparing IABP (n = 20) and TandemHeart pLVAD (n =21) in patients with revascularized MI complicated with cardiogenic shock, patients supported with pLVAD had better hemodynamics and metabolic variables compared with IABP; however, mortality was similar and there were more bleeding and vascular complications associated with pLVAD.[25] These results were replicated in another small randomized trial.[26] Despite the feasibility of this mode of circulatory support described in retrospective studies, along with the superior hemodynamic support compared with IABP, the clinical benefit of this device has not been established for use in patients undergoing HR-PCI. In experienced centers, HR-PCI can successfully be accomplished with low procedural complications.

The Impella

The Impella Circulatory Support System (Abiomed, Danvers, MA) is a different type of pLVAD that uses an Archimedes screw mechanism for LV unloading and circulatory assist. It consists of a miniature axial flow rotary blood pump that is positioned across the aortic valve (**Fig. 3**). The system actively unloads the ventricle by drawing blood through the distal port within the ventricular cavity and pumping it into the ascending aorta through the proximal port of the device. The inflow cannula pump is inserted via the femoral artery and advanced past the aortic valve under fluoroscopic guidance (see **Fig. 3**), which is the main difference with the TandemHeart (see **Table 1**). The Impella system provides in-parallel LV to aortic circulatory support, instead of LA to aortic.[15] This device is designed to provide short-term ventricular support for several hours to days and comes in 3 different sizes: the Impella system LP 2.5, CP, and 5.0, with 12-French, 14-French, and 21-French diameter pumps capable of providing flows of 2.5, around 4.0, and 5.0 L/min respectively. All systems are mounted on a 9-French pigtail catheter.[30] There are percutaneous (LP) and surgical implantable versions (LD) as well as a surgical implantable Impella for right ventricular support (RD). The device used for HR-PCI is almost exclusively the LP version. Although the femoral artery is the most common access, a right axillary approach has been used intraoperatively for postcardiotomy shock in patients with severe peripheral arterial disease.[31] A new-generation percutaneous device, the Impella CP, is capable of delivering up to 4 L/min of flow with an upgraded 14-French diameter pump, using the same console and 9-French pigtail catheter.

The Impella system received FDA approval in 2006 for up to 5-day support. Despite the transaortic-valve nature of the pump, no valvular damage has been reported and it has a good safety record when used up to 3 days.[32] Although there are some reports of successful bridge to recovery after acute myocarditis[33] and it has been studied in post-MI cardiogenic shock,[34,35] the most common use of this device to date is for patients undergoing HR-PCI.[4,5,36]

Implantation and device description The Impella system LP 2.5 and CP models are suited for percutaneous implantation, whereas the LP 5.0 model requires surgical cut-down of the femoral artery for insertion. Insertion is straightforward and can be learned readily by all interventional cardiologists. When the percutaneous system is used, a 13-French or 14-French sheath is placed into the

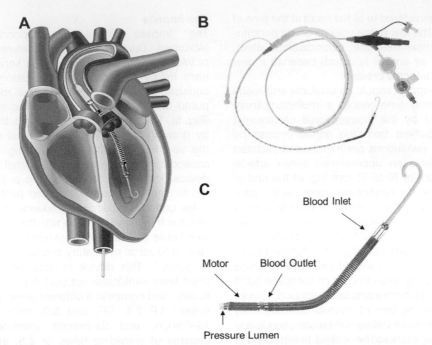

Fig. 3. The Impella LP circulatory support system (Abiomed, Danvers, MA). (*A*) Appropriate placement of the Impella Recover LP 2.5 device through the aortic valve into the left ventricle. (*B*) The Impella 2.5 system components. (*C*) The miniaturized pump. (*Courtesy of* Abiomed Inc., Danvers, MA; with permission.)

femoral artery using the Seldinger technique. A 5-French pigtail catheter is subsequently used to access the ventricle in a retrograde fashion. This catheter is then exchanged over a wire for the 12-French catheter-pump assembly and, once confirmed position in the LV cavity, circulatory support is initiated and titrated using the 9 different performance levels (P1–9, maximal flow of 2.5 vs around 4.0 L/min). Proper placement should be confirmed before initiation. The hinge of the Impella system should be placed at the level of the aortic valve.

The Impella system consists of the following components:

- Impella catheter with built-in pump
- Impella controller with portable battery
- Power supply and cable

Maintenance and explantation Systemic anticoagulation is necessary to reduce the risk of thromboembolic complications. After an ACT of 250 to 500 seconds is achieved, the device is inserted as described earlier. The ACT should be maintained at 160 to 180 seconds after device insertion and throughout circulatory support. A unique feature of this device is the integrated purge system that delivers 20% dextrose plus heparin 50 IU/mL to the Impella pump. Two weaning protocols have been described by the manufacturer; however, physician discretion and institutional

driven protocols may be used. The rapid weaning protocol consists of decreasing the performance level in 2-level steps every several minutes until level P2 is reached. This method is usually the preferred way of weaning after support for HR-PCI. The circulatory support should be maintained at this level for at least 10 minutes before discontinuing the device. After this interval, if the patient remains stable, the performance level is decreased to P1, the catheter is pulled back into the aortic root, and the pump is stopped. The catheter-pump is subsequently explanted and a percutaneous arterial closer is usually needed.

When supporting patients with cardiogenic shock, the slow weaning protocol may be more appropriate. This protocol is achieved by decreasing the pump performance by 2 levels at 2-hour to 3-hour intervals. Caution is needed to avoid decreasing the pump performance level to less than P2 while the catheter is in the ventricle because retrograde flow may occur. Once the patient is stable on performance level P2 for at least 2 hours, the performance level is reduce to P1 and the catheter is pulled back to the aorta to subsequently stop the pump. After discontinuation of heparin and ACT less than 150 seconds, the cannula is removed as previously described.

Contraindications The Impella is contraindicated in the presence of a prosthetic aortic valve because of risk of damage to the prosthetic leaflets, a severely calcified aortic valve with or without aortic stenosis, significant aortic regurgitation (grade 2 or more), presence of LV thrombus, VSD, and severe peripheral arterial disease. Other relative contraindications include abdominal or thoracoabdominal aortic aneurysms, aortic dissection, and the presence of femoral-popliteal bypass grafts. The use in the presence of aortobifemoral grafts has never been described, and should be discussed with a vascular surgeon if used for elective circulatory support. However, the axillary or subclavian artery approach has been used and could be considered in this patient population.[37]

Complications and limitations Potential complications of the Impella include cerebral vascular accident, aortic valve injury with resultant aortic insufficiency, arrhythmia (atrial and ventricular), cardiac tamponade, infection, vascular injury, limb ischemia, bleeding, and coagulopathy.

This device can also provoke hemolysis and thrombocytopenia.[38] This finding is usually not clinically significant and rarely requires transfusion or termination of the device. Vascular and bleeding complications seem to be comparable with IABP compared with the IABP.[39] Although the use of this device has gained significant popularity for temporary circulatory support for cardiogenic shock and HR-PCI, because of the obviation of concomitant venous cannulation and transseptal puncture, the hemodynamic response to the device is variable and occasionally can cause LV volume overload.[40,41] This phenomenon could be related to malpositioning of the pump (too deep) or peridevice leak limiting proper coaptation of the aortic valve leaflets. Furthermore, there is a well-documented learning curve for the use of this device.[5]

Role of the Impella system in HR-PCI The Impella pLVAD has the advantage of not requiring venous access and transseptal puncture, and has gained significant popularity in these patients. The new Impella CP is capable of providing up to around 4 L/min of support, and has created opportunities for patients undergoing HR-PCI and in cardiogenic shock. The complication rate is comparable with the IABP[39] and may be more cost-effective.[42]

Multiple studies have shown the feasibility of the Impella system for patients undergoing HR-PCI and to support cardiogenic shock.[36,43,44]

The USpella registry[4] is a prospective registry for patients receiving hemodynamic support with the Impella 2.5 device. This study showed a

significant increase in LV ejection fraction (LVEF) after hemodynamically supported HR-PCI, with improvement in functional status, reduction of implantable cardioverter defibrillator target population, and low mortality with low rate of major adverse cardiac events (MACE) compared with the known HR-PCI literature.

The ISAR-SHOCK, was a small randomized controlled trial that compared the Impella 2.5 (n = 12) with the IABP (n = 13) in patients with cardiogenic shock after acute MI.[34] The primary end point was the change in cardiac index from baseline to 30 minutes after implantation. Although the Impella 2.5 resulted in a greater increase in cardiac index compared with the IABP at 30 minutes (Impella change in Cardiac Index [ΔCI] = 0.49 $\pm$ 0.46 L/min/m^2; IABP, ΔCI = 0.11 $\pm$ 0.31 L/min/m^2; P = .02). Nevertheless, the difference disappeared at all other time points up to 30 hours. Mortality was similar between the groups. This study showed that the use of the Impella to support patients in cardiogenic shock was feasible and provided faster hemodynamic stabilization, despite the effects not being sustained at 30 hours.

With the premise that the Impella provides superior ventricular support compared with the IABP, the PROTECT II (A Prospective, Multi-center, Randomized Controlled Trial of the IMPELLA RECOVER LP 2.5 System Versus Intra-Aortic Balloon Pump (IABP) in Patients Undergoing Non Emergent High Risk PCI) trial investigators performed the first FDA-approved, prospective, multi-center study for patients requiring hemodynamic support during HR-PCI, comparing the effectiveness and outcomes between the IABP and Impella 2.5.[5] The criteria for HR-PCI were the presence of unprotected left main coronary artery disease and LVEF less than 30%. The primary end point was the 30-day incidence of major adverse events (MAE). MAEs included all-cause mortality, acute MI, stroke, repeat revascularization, acute kidney injury, severe intraprocedural hypotension, cardiopulmonary resuscitation, aortic insufficiency, and angiographic failure of PCI. The trial was terminated by the data and safety monitoring board because of futility. Any subsequent post hoc analyses are, at best, speculative but do suggest potential fruitful future areas of investigation. The scientific merit of a prespecified analysis in a prematurely discontinued study should be seen as hypothesis generating because the study did not meet the primary end point. The following statement should therefore be evaluated in this context. Although there was no difference in MAE at 30 days, the Impella arm had strong trends toward superior clinical outcomes for the intent-to-treat population, with a significant reduction of the MAE rate in the prespecified protocol population at 90 days. The Impella also showed superior hemodynamic support as measured by the cardiac power output. The treatment effect of Impella compared with IABP improved over the course of the trial, suggesting a learning curve. The clinical benefit was more pronounced for patients undergoing HR-PCI without atherectomy with the Impella support. This trial showed the noninferiority of the Impella 2.5 compared with IABP for hemodynamic support in patients undergoing HR-PCI. As improved pumps with fewer adverse effects and improved support, such as the Impella CP, arrive, more data will be required in randomized trials or prospective registries to validate the use of this device in patients undergoing HR-PCI as well as in patients with cardiogenic shock.

ECMO

Although, in theory, ECMO qualifies as percutaneous circulatory support, its role in HR-PCI is limited to emergent and rescue use in severe cardiopulmonary failure. The previously described pLVADs depend on satisfactory lung function to provide adequate systemic support. ECMO consists of a blood pump and a circuit with a built-in oxygenator, with the capability to provide partial to near-full cardiopulmonary support. Although there are different cannulation routes, the classic percutaneous access for adults in cardiopulmonary collapse is achieved via femoral vessels to provide venous-arterial bypass. Venovenous ECMO via a transjugular approach with a dual-lumen single cannula can be used for respiratory failure alone.

In adults, a 16-French to 18-French arterial cannula is inserted via the femoral artery into the descending aorta and an 18-French to 20-French venous cannula inserted via the contralateral femoral vein into the right atrium. After appropriate deairing, these cannulas are connected to the external pump and membrane oxygenator. The pump is primed with a crystalloid-colloid solution, and blood is subsequently withdrawn from the right atrium, pumped through the heat exchanger and membrane oxygenator, and returned via the femoral artery to the aorta. The circulatory support is retrograde continuous flow, but usually pulsatile arterial pressure is maintained unless ECMO is providing complete cardiopulmonary support. Limitations of ECMO in the catheterization laboratory include lack of direct LV unloading, increased LV afterload, and the requirement of more personnel (ECMO specialists, perfusionists). Furthermore, it produces a more pronounced systemic inflammatory response.[45] It requires the same level of anticoagulation as the previously described devices and concomitant intra-aortic counterpulsation can be used, especially in the context of myocardial ischemia. In the current era of partial circulatory support, the role of standard ECMO in the catheterization laboratory is limited to refractory cardiopulmonary failure in which percutaneous ventricular assistance alone is not sufficient because of concomitant respiratory failure. Moreover, this mode of circulatory support can be used to maintain homeostasis as bridge to emergent cardiac surgery.

Portable ECMO devices suited for transport and capable of full cardiopulmonary bypass, with easier use, have been developed and include the LIFEBRIDGE B2 T System (Medizintechnik GmbH, Ampfing, Germany)[46] and the CARDIOHELP (MAQUET Getinge Group, Hirrlingen, Germany) ECMO systems.[47]

PERSPECTIVE

The development of pLVADs has created opportunities for patients undergoing HR-PCI. As new studies are published establishing the role of these devices, it is important to understand the unique hemodynamic benefit that they provide. LV unloading with maintenance of systemic and coronary perfusion separates these devices from traditional IABP and ECMO support. Once an established learning curve has been achieved, it may account for important difference in patient outcomes, not only in HR-PCI but in cardiogenic shock. These devices are likely to play an important role in the management of high-risk patients, although the indications and contraindications for their use are still evolving. The role of a pLVAD in HR-PCI has become limited because, even in patients previously thought to be high risk, the procedure can be done safely without support. The high-risk patient (poor LV function) with a high-risk lesion would be the patient most likely to benefit from PCI performed with pLVAD support.

REFERENCES

1. Bounous EP, Mark DB, Pollock BG, et al. Surgical survival benefits for coronary disease patients with left ventricular dysfunction. Circulation 1988;78(3 Pt 2):I151–7.
2. Remmelink M, Sjauw KD, Henriques JP, et al. Effects of mechanical left ventricular unloading by Impella on left ventricular dynamics in high-risk and primary percutaneous coronary intervention patients. Cather Cardiovasc Interv 2010;75(2):187–94.

3. Alli OO, Singh IM, Holmes DR Jr, et al. Percutaneous left ventricular assist device with TandemHeart for high-risk percutaneous coronary intervention: the Mayo Clinic experience. Catheter Cardiovasc Interv 2012;80(5):728–34.

4. Maini B, Naidu SS, Mulukutla S, et al. Real-world use of the Impella 2.5 circulatory support system in complex high-risk percutaneous coronary intervention: the USpella Registry. Catheter Cardiovasc Interv 2012;80(5):717–25.

5. O'Neill WW, Kleiman NS, Moses J, et al. A prospective, randomized clinical trial of hemodynamic support with Impella 2.5 versus intra-aortic balloon pump in patients undergoing high-risk percutaneous coronary intervention: the PROTECT II Study. Circulation 2012;126(14):1717–27.

6. Antman EM, Anbe DT, Armstrong PW, et al. ACC/AHA guidelines for the management of patients with ST-elevation myocardial infarction–executive summary. A report of the American College of Cardiology/American Heart Association Task Force on Practice Guidelines (Writing Committee to revise the 1999 guidelines for the management of patients with acute myocardial infarction). J Am Coll Cardiol 2004;44(3):671–719.

7. Levine GN, Bates ER, Blankenship JC, et al. 2011 ACCF/AHA/SCAI guideline for percutaneous coronary intervention. A report of the American College of Cardiology Foundation/American Heart Association Task Force on Practice Guidelines and the Society for Cardiovascular Angiography and Interventions. J Am Coll Cardiol 2011;58(24):e44–122.

8. Bregman D, Casarella WJ. Percutaneous intraaortic balloon pumping: initial clinical experience. Ann Thorac Surg 1980;29(2):153–5.

9. Stone GW, Ohman EM, Miller MF, et al. Contemporary utilization and outcomes of intra-aortic balloon counterpulsation in acute myocardial infarction: the benchmark registry. J Am Coll Cardiol 2003;41(11):1940–5.

10. Ferguson JJ 3rd, Cohen M, Freedman RJ Jr, et al. The current practice of intra-aortic balloon counterpulsation: results from the Benchmark Registry. J Am Coll Cardiol 2001;38(5):1456–62.

11. Ishihara M, Sato H, Tateishi H, et al. Intraaortic balloon pumping as the postangioplasty strategy in acute myocardial infarction. Am Heart J 1991;122(2):385–9.

12. Perera D, Stables R, Thomas M, et al. Elective intra-aortic balloon counterpulsation during high-risk percutaneous coronary intervention: a randomized controlled trial. JAMA 2010;304(8):867–74.

13. Prondzinsky R, Lemm H, Swyter M, et al. Intra-aortic balloon counterpulsation in patients with acute myocardial infarction complicated by cardiogenic shock: the prospective, randomized IABP SHOCK Trial for attenuation of multiorgan dysfunction syndrome. Crit Care Med 2010;38(1):152–60.

14. Thiele H, Zeymer U, Neumann FJ, et al. Intraaortic balloon support for myocardial infarction with cardiogenic shock. N Engl J Med 2012;367(14):1287–96.

15. Naidu SS. Novel percutaneous cardiac assist devices: the science of and indications for hemodynamic support. Circulation 2011;123(5):533–43.

16. Thiele H, Smalling RW, Schuler GC. Percutaneous left ventricular assist devices in acute myocardial infarction complicated by cardiogenic shock. Eur Heart J 2007;28(17):2057–63.

17. Dennis C, Carlens E, Senning A, et al. Clinical use of a cannula for left heart bypass without thoracotomy: experimental protection against fibrillation by left heart bypass. Ann Surg 1962;156:623–37.

18. Glassman E, Chinitz LA, Levite HA, et al. Percutaneous left atrial to femoral arterial bypass pumping for circulatory support in high-risk coronary angioplasty. Cathet Cardiovasc Diagn 1993;29(3):210–6.

19. Aragon J, Lee MS, Kar S, et al. Percutaneous left ventricular assist device: "TandemHeart" for high-risk coronary intervention. Catheter Cardiovasc Interv 2005;65(3):346–52.

20. Vranckx P, Meliga E, De Jaegere PP, et al. The TandemHeart, percutaneous transseptal left ventricular assist device: a safeguard in high-risk percutaneous coronary interventions. The six-year Rotterdam experience. EuroIntervention 2008;4(3):331–7.

21. Atiemo AD, Conte JV, Heldman AW. Resuscitation and recovery from acute right ventricular failure using a percutaneous right ventricular assist device. Catheter Cardiovasc Interv 2006;68(1):78–82.

22. Prutkin JM, Strote JA, Stout KK. Percutaneous right ventricular assist device as support for cardiogenic shock due to right ventricular infarction. J Invasive Cardiol 2008;20(7):E215–6.

23. Chiam PT, Ruiz CE, Cohen HA. Placement of a large transseptal cannula through an inferior vena cava filter for TandemHeart percutaneous left ventricular assist. J Invasive Cardiol 2008;20(6):E197–9.

24. Thiele H, Lauer B, Hambrecht R, et al. Reversal of cardiogenic shock by percutaneous left atrial-to-femoral arterial bypass assistance. Circulation 2001;104(24):2917–22.

25. Thiele H, Sick P, Boudriot E, et al. Randomized comparison of intra-aortic balloon support with a percutaneous left ventricular assist device in patients with revascularized acute myocardial infarction complicated by cardiogenic shock. Eur Heart J 2005;26(13):1276–83.

26. Burkhoff D, Cohen H, Brunckhorst C, et al. A randomized multicenter clinical study to evaluate the safety and efficacy of the TandemHeart percutaneous ventricular assist device versus conventional therapy with intraaortic balloon pumping for

treatment of cardiogenic shock. Am Heart J 2006; 152(3):469.e1–8.

27. Vranckx P, Schultz CJ, Valgimigli M, et al. Assisted circulation using the TandemHeart during very high-risk PCI of the unprotected left main coronary artery in patients declined for CABG. Catheter Cardiovasc Interv 2009;74(2):302–10.

28. Schwartz BG, Ludeman DJ, Mayeda GS, et al. High-risk percutaneous coronary intervention with the TandemHeart and Impella devices: a single-center experience. J Invasive Cardiol 2011;23(10):417–24.

29. Tempelhof MW, Klein L, Cotts WG, et al. Clinical experience and patient outcomes associated with the TandemHeart percutaneous transseptal assist device among a heterogeneous patient population. ASAIO J 2011;57(4):254–61.

30. Garatti A, Colombo T, Russo C, et al. Left ventricular mechanical support with the Impella Recover left direct microaxial blood pump: a single-center experience. Artif Organs 2006;30(7):523–8.

31. Sassard T, Scalabre A, Bonnefoy E, et al. The right axillary artery approach for the Impella Recover LP 5.0 microaxial pump. Ann Thorac Surg 2008;85(4): 1468–70.

32. Engstrom AE, Sjauw KD, Baan J, et al. Long-term safety and sustained left ventricular recovery: long-term results of percutaneous left ventricular support with Impella LP2.5 in ST-elevation myocardial infarction. EuroIntervention 2011;6(7):860–5.

33. Colombo T, Garatti A, Bruschi G, et al. First successful bridge to recovery with the Impella Recover 100 left ventricular assist device for fulminant acute myocarditis. Ital Heart J 2003;4(9):642–5.

34. Seyfarth M, Sibbing D, Bauer I, et al. A randomized clinical trial to evaluate the safety and efficacy of a percutaneous left ventricular assist device versus intra-aortic balloon pumping for treatment of cardiogenic shock caused by myocardial infarction. J Am Coll Cardiol 2008;52(19):1584–8.

35. Cheng JM, den Uil CA, Hoeks SE, et al. Percutaneous left ventricular assist devices vs. intra-aortic balloon pump counterpulsation for treatment of cardiogenic shock: a meta-analysis of controlled trials. Eur Heart J 2009;30(17):2102–8.

36. Henriques JP, Remmelink M, Baan J Jr, et al. Safety and feasibility of elective high-risk percutaneous coronary intervention procedures with left ventricular support of the Impella Recover LP 2.5. Am J Cardiol 2006;97(7):990–2.

37. Lotun K, Shetty R, Patel M, et al. Percutaneous left axillary artery approach for Impella 2.5 liter

circulatory support for patients with severe aortoiliac arterial disease undergoing high-risk percutaneous coronary intervention. J Interv Cardiol 2012;25(2): 210–3.

38. Meyns B, Dens J, Sergeant P, et al. Initial experiences with the Impella device in patients with cardiogenic shock - Impella support for cardiogenic shock. Thorac Cardiovasc Surg 2003;51(6): 312–7.

39. Boudoulas KD, Pederzolli A, Saini U, et al. Comparison of Impella and intra-aortic balloon pump in high-risk percutaneous coronary intervention: vascular complications and incidence of bleeding. Acute Card Care 2012;14(4):120–4.

40. Valgimigli M, Steendijk P, Serruys PW, et al. Use of Impella Recover(R) LP 2.5 left ventricular assist device during high-risk percutaneous coronary interventions; clinical, haemodynamic and biochemical findings. EuroIntervention 2006;2(1):91–100.

41. Thomopoulou S, Manginas A, Cokkinos DV. Initial experience with the Impella Recover LP 2.5 micro-axial pump in patients undergoing high-risk coronary angioplasty. Hellenic J Cardiol 2008;49(6): 382–7.

42. Roos JB, Doshi SN, Konorza T, et al. The cost-effectiveness of a new percutaneous ventricular assist device for high-risk PCI patients: mid-stage evaluation from the European perspective. J Med Econ 2013;16(3):381–90.

43. Dixon SR, Henriques JP, Mauri L, et al. A prospective feasibility trial investigating the use of the Impella 2.5 system in patients undergoing high-risk percutaneous coronary intervention (The PROTECT I Trial): initial U.S. experience. JACC Cardiovasc Interv 2009;2(2):91–6.

44. Burzotta F, Paloscia L, Trani C, et al. Feasibility and long-term safety of elective Impella-assisted high-risk percutaneous coronary intervention: a pilot two-centre study. J Cardiovasc Med (Hagerstown) 2008;9(10):1004–10.

45. Kale P, Fang JC. Devices in acute heart failure. Crit Care Med 2008;36(Suppl 1):S121–8.

46. Buz S, Jurmann MJ, Gutsch E, et al. Portable mechanical circulatory support: human experience with the LIFEBRIDGE system. Ann Thorac Surg 2011;91(5):1591–5.

47. Arlt M, Philipp A, Voelkel S, et al. Hand-held mini-mised extracorporeal membrane oxygenation: a new bridge to recovery in patients with out-of-centre cardiogenic shock. Eur J Cardiothorac Surg 2011;40(3):689–94.

Percutaneous Assist Device for Cardiopulmonary Resuscitation

Vegard Tuseth, MD, PhD[a,b,*]

KEYWORDS

- Cardiopulmonary resuscitation • Percutaneous assist device • Cardiac arrest
- Ventricular fibrillation

KEY POINTS

- Cardiac arrest still has a very poor prognosis if the initial defibrillation is unsuccessful.
- Current treatment algorithms are under debate.
- Cardiac arrest is most often caused by coronary ischemia.
- Emergency use of mechanical hemodynamic support and coronary revascularization may have the potential to improve results.
- Impella percutaneous left ventricular assist devices offer an attractive approach for use in the catheterization laboratory in this setting.

INTRODUCTION

Cardiac arrest is defined as sudden circulatory collapse with loss of consciousness and absent arterial pulses. Cardiac arrest can result from a broad spectrum of medical conditions as well as primary cardiac disorders.[1,2]

Incidence

The incidence of out-of-hospital cardiac arrest treated by emergency medical services (EMS) was 56 per 100 000 in a recent study of cardiac arrest in the Bergen region. This incidence is in line with previous national studies (37–60 per 100 000) and international studies (38–65 per 100 000).[3,4] In this study, 64% had a probable cardiac cause, of which ischemic events constitute the most.[5] Data from the author's hospital showed that only one-third of patients with cardiac arrest presented with shockable rhythms (ventricular fibrillation [VF] or ventricular tachycardia [VT]), whereas two-thirds presented with nonshockable rhythms, such as asystole, pulseless electrical activity, and bradycardia.

Prognosis

Shockable rhythm (VF, VT) is a major predictor of survival.[3,6,7] Furthermore, survival is improved by specific treatment algorithms, including trained prehospital and in-hospital teams and equipment. Algorithms, such as "Chain-of-survival,"[1] include early warning, early cardiopulmonary resuscitation (CPR), early defibrillation, and postresuscitation care including hypothermia.[8–10] Other predictors of outcome are the duration of cardiac standstill and the presence of an acute reversible underlying cause of hemodynamic collapse.[10,11] Thus, although the prognosis is generally poor in cardiac arrest, clinical factors, including presenting rhythm, quality and speed of advanced cardiac life support (ACLS), and cause, are considered critical predictors for successful restoration of spontaneous circulation (ROSC) with current treatment.[12,13] However, recently the benefits of parts of these generally accepted algorithms have been questioned. Algorithms are complex and, to some extent, based on empiric and experimental data. Further clinical research aims to further assess the usefulness of established treatment,

[a] Department of Heart Disease, Haukeland University Hospital, Bergen 5021, Norway; [b] K2 Department, Institute of Internal Medicine, University of Bergen, Jonas Lies vei, Bergen 5021, Norway
* Department of Heart Disease, Haukeland University Hospital, Bergen 5021, Norway.
E-mail address: Vegard.Tuseth@helse-bergen.no

Intervent Cardiol Clin 2 (2013) 429–443
http://dx.doi.org/10.1016/j.iccl.2013.03.003
2211-7458/13/$ – see front matter © 2013 Elsevier Inc. All rights reserved.

including adrenaline, chest compressions, and hypothermia. Novel approaches may be needed to improve treatment in cardiac arrest (**Fig. 1**).

Coronary Ischemia

Coronary ischemia is the most frequent cause of cardiac arrest.[3,14] Acute percutaneous coronary intervention (PCI) may improve prognosis for patients with ST-elevation myocardial infarction after a successful initial resuscitation.[15,16] However, most patients with cardiac arrest admitted to the hospital after ROSC do not present with ST elevation, and the prognostic benefit of acute revascularization in such patients has not been established (**Table 1**).

Persistent Cardiac Arrest

Patients who do not achieve ROSC in a prehospital setting are only rarely transported to the hospital and have an extremely poor prognosis.[17,18] In patients without reestablishment of spontaneous cardiac function after 3 cycles of ACLS

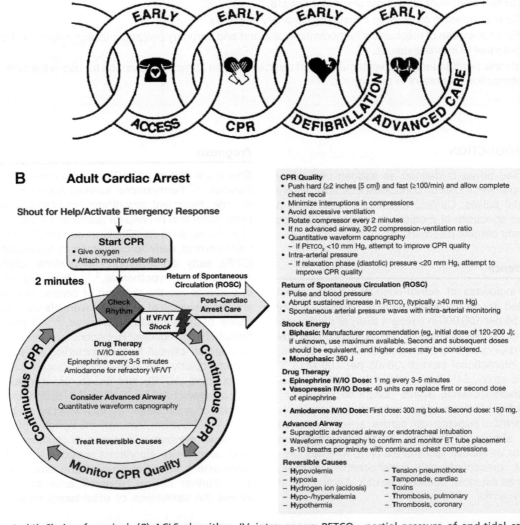

Fig. 1. (*A*) Chain of survival. (*B*) ACLS algorithm. IV, intravenous; PETCO₂, partial pressure of end-tidal carbon dioxide. ET, End Tidal; IO, Intra Osseous. (*From* [A] Cummins RO, Ornato JP, Thies WH, et al. Improving survival from sudden cardiac arrest: the "chain of survival" concept. A statement for health professionals from the Advanced Cardiac Life Support Subcommittee and the Emergency Cardiac Care Committee, American Heart Association. Circulation 1991;83:1832–47; with permission; [B] Neumar RW, Otto CW, Link MS, et al. Part 8: adult advanced cardiovascular life support: 2010 American Heart Association guidelines for cardiopulmonary resuscitation and emergency cardiovascular care. Circulation 2010;122:S729–67; with permission.)

Table 1
Angiographic data in the 84 patients who underwent angiography[a]

Variable	Value
Normal coronary arteries: No. (%)	17 (20)
Clinically insignificant coronary artery disease ($\leq$50% stenosis): No. (%)	7 (8)
Clinically significant coronary artery disease: No. (%)	60 (71)
Single-vessel disease	22
2-vessel disease	13
3-vessel disease	24
Isolated left main coronary artery disease	1
Left ventricular ejection fraction (%)	33.9 ± 10.5
Left ventricular end-diastolic pressure (mm Hg)	25.3 ± 9.5

[a] Plus/minus values are means ± standard deviation. Because of rounding, the percentages do not total 100.
   Data from Spaulding CM, Joly LM, Rosenberg A, et al. Immediate coronary angiography in survivors of out-of-hospital cardiac arrest. N Engl J Med 1997;336(23): 1629–33.

(approximately 10 minutes of treatment), survival is rare both in and out of the hospital. In this setting with persistent cardiac arrest, vital organ perfusion is poor and irreversible cardiac and cerebral damage is likely to occur rapidly.

This far, no adjunctive treatment has been able to consistently improve survival in such cases of refractory persistent cardiac arrest. However, sporadic cases have been reported with likely survival benefit with invasive hemodynamic support and revascularization in addition to conventional CPR in this setting (**Box 1**). Also, urgent cardio-pulmonary bypass, sophisticated resuscitation techniques, and medical adjunctive therapy have been studied but have not resulted in consistently better outcomes in clinical practice. Generally, survival remains near zero for such patients, but novel approaches give hope for improvement (**Fig. 2**).

Current Treatment Options

Acute revascularization with PCI can be performed with some technical difficulty during ongoing chest compressions.[19] Limited data indicate the feasibility of continued advanced hemodynamic support combined with acute coronary revascularization in selected cases.[20]

However, any reliable clinical benefit of such treatment has not been proven. In today's practice,

Box 1
Potential to improve current treatment

- Cardiac arrest is mainly caused by coronary ischemia.
- There are poor results with optimal current treatment.
- Persistent cardiac arrest has almost 100% mortality.
- Emergency revascularization and hemodynamic support could be lifesaving.

ACLS is most commonly performed until ROSC or death and very few patients are transported to hospital during on-going resuscitation.

Optimal revascularization during on-going chest compressions is complicated in clinical practice and suboptimal performance may have detrimental effects on outcomes. Current routine practice does not include emergency PCI or cardiac assist therapy.

Causes of Persistent Cardiac Arrest

In persistent cardiac arrest, on-going coronary ischemia may impair the effect of CPR and defibrillation. Stenosis or occlusion of major coronary

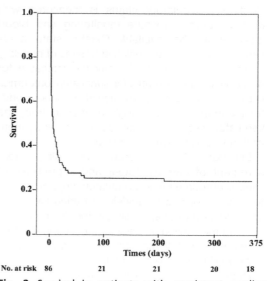

Fig. 2. Survival in patients with persistent cardiac arrest treated with extracorporeal membrane oxygenation plus PCI. (*From* Kagawa E, Dote K, Kato M, et al. Should we emergently revascularize occluded coronaries for cardiac arrest?: rapid-response extracorporeal membrane oxygenation and intra-arrest percutaneous coronary intervention. Circulation 2012; 126:1605–13; with permission.)

vessels may cause ischemic myocardial damage with substantial areas of electrical instability. In turn, this can maintain VF or conduction abnormalities refractory to defibrillation.[21,22]

Sustained myocardial hypoperfusion causes interstitial hyperkalemia, acidosis, and activation of reactive oxygen species.[23] During ischemia, depletion of cellular energy stores and mitochondrial dysfunction can induce disruption of cardiomyocyte membrane stability.[24] All of these mechanisms could, in theory, be relieved by reperfusion therapy. However, in clinical practice, urgent revascularization is often not enough to stabilize patients.

Possibly, reperfusion needs to be maintained beyond the initial phase including reperfusion injury to have an optimal stabilizing effect.

Data during chest compressions suggest that increased intraventricular pressures may impair coronary perfusion, which can further reduce the chances of successful defibrillation.[25] Left ventricular pressures may be effectively modified by cardiac assist therapy.[26] Lowering intraventricular pressures and increasing coronary perfusion with a mechanical hemodynamic assist device could facilitate myocardial blood flow and reduce the likelihood of refractory arrhythmia.

Prognostic Assessment in Persistent Cardiac Arrest

Routinely, circulatory status is monitored with invasive blood pressure monitoring and blood gas analysis when available. Cerebral status is assessed clinically often using estimates of pupillary reaction. These methods may be unreliable for determining the potential for successful outcomes in this complex setting. The use of continuous end-tidal carbon dioxide (CO_2) monitoring from the ventilator requires minor additional equipment and may add relevant information.

End-tidal CO_2 monitoring is an indirect measurement of cardiac output and a predictor of clinical outcomes when ventilatory support is performed according to guidelines during CPR.[27–29] This monitoring offers a simple tool for better assessing the clinical efficacy of conventional resuscitation and for left ventricular assist device (LVAD) support during cardiac arrest.

High values are associated with improved systemic, cerebral, and myocardial circulation and may identify patients when further intervention can be implemented with potential to improve survival.[30] Very low values can be used to predict death in prolonged resuscitation.[31] Similar correlations have been found in experimental studies of percutaneous LVAD support during VF (**Fig. 3**).[32]

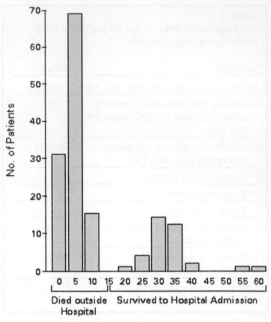

Fig. 3. End-tidal CO_2 level. (*From* Levine RL, Wayne MA, Miller CC. End-tidal carbon dioxide and outcome of out-of-hospital cardiac arrest. N Engl J Med 1997;337:301–6. Copyright © 1997 Massachusetts Medical Society. *Reprinted* with permission from Massachusetts Medical Society.)

Medical Intervention

Vasopressors and antiarrhythmic drugs intuitively could be useful in addition to chest compressions in the setting of persistent cardiac arrest. Several substances have been used, but effects on survival have not been found.

Currently, routine use of intravenous adrenaline is recommended in current guidelines.[1] However, adrenalinelike substances may have detrimental circulatory and metabolic effects in persistent ischemic cardiac arrest despite the intuitive benefit of increased arterial pressures. Experimentally, both cerebral and coronary perfusion have been shown to be impaired with the use of vasopressor therapy during cardiac arrest.[33,34] A lack of benefit and possible adverse effects have also been indicated on clinical outcomes in resuscitation.[35,36] Also, intravenous amiodarone is considered in current guidelines.[1] This potent antiarrhythmic drug has been shown to improve out-of-hospital ROSC but has not had any effect on survival to hospital discharge after cardiac arrest. The possible reasons for drugs like amiodarone and adrenaline being effective on ROSC but not on survival to discharge are still unclear. It cannot be ruled out that unrecognized adverse clinical effects may out weigh the beneficial effects on the short-term cardiac rhythm. However, the use of low-dose norepinephrine is recommended to counteract vasodilatation in patients on Impella (Abiomed, Danvers, MA) treatment (**Fig. 4**).

CPR Devices

The use of mechanical compression-decompression devices has been shown to be hemodynamically effective in experimental studies but has as of yet failed to prove a definitive clinical advantage compared with manual chest compressions in cardiac arrest.[37–40] Abdominal compression either manually or with specific devices can have a hemodynamic benefit (**Fig. 5**).

Surgically Implanted LVADs

LVADs are established treatment choices in chronic heart failure and reduced left ventricular workload and oxygen consumption, with possible beneficial effects on myocardial metabolism and function.[41–44] Surgical LVADs have been implanted successfully in shock and in cardiac arrest and may be useful as a bridge to permanent treatment or recovery for selected patients after initial stabilization.[45]

Surgically implanted LVADs provide systemic blood delivery and myocardial unloading in severe

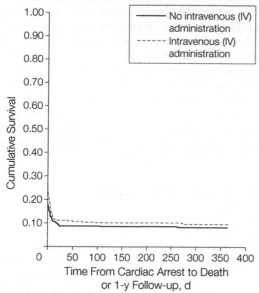

Fig. 4. Survival after cardiac arrest with and without intravenous medical therapy. (*From* Olasveengen TM, Sunde K, Brunborg C, et al. Intravenous drug administration during out-of-hospital cardiac arrest: a randomized trial. JAMA 2009;302(20):2222–9; with permission. Copyright © 2009 American Medical Association. All rights reserved.)

heart failure, including the acute setting, and have been proven clinically effective for long-term use in chronic heart failure.[46]

Mechanical assist devices could, in theory, facilitate revascularization and also improve vital organ perfusion during cardiac arrest.

Acute surgical implantation has a high risk of complications and requires highly specialized personnel and facilities. Thus, acute surgical LVAD support is not routinely available in the treatment of critical heart failure, and technical limitations may represent a substantial drawback in an acute critical setting.

Cardiopulmonary Support

Available cardiopulmonary support (CPS) systems also include cardiopulmonary bypass (CPB) and extracorporeal membrane oxygenation (ECMO) and extracorporeal life support (ECLS), which have the potential to sustain circulation during cardiac standstill.

Reports on the use of ECMO, ECLS, and CPB in cardiogenic shock and cardiac arrest have shown the feasibility of such interventions, but a potential to improve survival in a routine clinical setting has not been established.[47–49] Particularly, results with ECMO have been favorable in the treatment of refractory cardiac arrest, with survival rates between 30% and 40% in nonrandomized registries.[46,50] Furthermore, recent data also suggest improved survival rates in patients with acute myocardial infarction (AMI) and refractory shock with sophisticated algorithms with a combination of percutaneous ECMO, intra-aortic balloon pump (IABP), and low-dose inotropic support.[51]

ECMO may have the potential to restore circulation in persistent cardiac arrest and sustain circulation in patients with severe shock after ROSC.

Thus, it seems likely that hemodynamic support with ECMO, potentially in combination with additional support devices, may have lifesaving potential in persistent cardiac arrest.

A major issue limiting the practical use of CPS systems in cardiac arrest includes the complex logistic and technical procedures required during preparation, implantation, and follow-up.

A theoretical limitation for the successful use of ECMO in patients with AMI is the lack of left ventricular unloading, which may impair myocardial recovery in this setting. This limitation may be overcome with the simultaneous use of additional mechanical unloading with IABP or possibly Impella devices (**Box 2**).

Ideally, implantation should be rapid and uncomplicated and should not infer with on-going chest compressions or delay emergency coronary

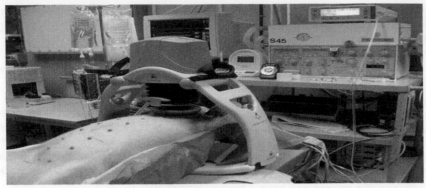

Fig. 5. Lukas mechanical chest compression-decompression device (Jolife AB, Lund, Sweden) mounted on a pig. LUCAS provides automatic mechanical compression and active decompression but only returning to the neutral position of the chest, with a frequency of 100 min. (*From* Rubertsson S, Karlsten R. Increased cortical cerebral blood flow with LUCAS: a new device for mechanical chest compressions compared to standard external compressions during experimental cardiopulmonary resuscitation. Resuscitation 2005;65(3):357–63; with permission.)

revascularization when required. Devices with reduced time of deployment and lower risk of complications could further improve results with mechanical hemodynamic support during cardiac arrest (**Fig. 6**).

Percutaneous LVADs

Newly developed percutaneous LVADs (PVADs) have the advantage of relatively rapid and simple deployment compared with CPS and surgical LVADs. Safety and feasibility for short-term clinical use have been established. Available devices include Impella devices and TandemHeart (Cardiac assist, Pittsburg, PA). These devices have been assessed in AMI, cardiogenic shock, severe heart failure, high-risk PCI, and as a bridge to permanent treatment in decompensated heart failure.

Furthermore, limited clinical data suggest a possible benefit with the Impella 2.5 in patients undergoing PCI and also during AMI.[50,52,53] The device has also been used as bridge therapy in

terminal decompensated heart failure.[54] In patients being treated for ischemic cardiac arrest, the use of PVAD support may be beneficial by providing left ventricular unloading during and after ischemic myocardial injury as well as by improving cardiac and cerebral circulation. With a more physiologic blood flow pattern and improved unloading of the left ventricle, intraventricular impeller devices theoretically could be superior to other approaches in this setting. Increased output and unloading with larger Impella 5.0 LP devices may have theoretic advantages. Because of the more complicated surgical implantation that may complicate implantation in the acute setting, the 5.0 is often used in selected cases as a follow-up device after the initial treatment with the smaller device. The novel Impella CP can give up to 4-L blood delivery with a 14F percutaneous insertion and may represent the currently best compromise between size and delivery for most patients.

Resuscitation Versus Severe Cardiogenic Shock

Despite promising hemodynamic and clinical data for percutaneous LVAD support in cardiogenic shock, the potential use of such devices in persistent cardiac arrest remains uncertain and the clinical experience is limited. During cardiac standstill, the required filling of the left ventricle from the right may be severely impaired. If sufficient circulation from the right to the left cannot be obtained, blood delivery from an LVAD pump will be limited and unlikely to sustain over time. Possibly, the simultaneous use of chest- or abdominal-compression devices as well as intravenous fluid loading can have an effect in such cases.

Box 2
Possible approaches

- Emergency PCI in persistent cardiac arrest is feasible.
- CPR devices may facilitate transport.
- Surgical LVAD is too complicated in the acute setting.
- ECMO has been used with promising effect.
- Impella permits more easy and physiologic support.

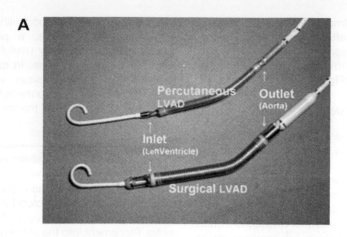

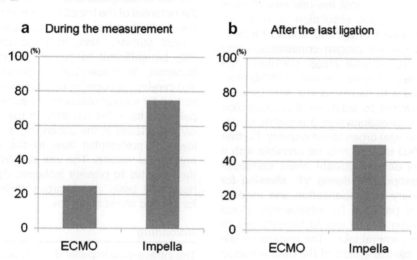

Fig. 6. (*A*) LVADs. The percutaneous LVAD (Impella LP 2.5) is on top, and the surgical LVAD (Impella LP 5.0) is on the bottom. (*B*) Successful defibrillation rate: number of successful defibrillated dogs/number of dogs who suffered from VF × 100 (%). (*a*) During the experiment (before the last left anterior descending coronary artery [LAD] ligation), VF occurred in 4 dogs. Although only one dog recovered heartbeats with direct cardioversion (DC) under ECMO support, the other 3 recovered heartbeats successfully with DC only under Impella support. (*b*) After the last LAD ligation, VF occurred in 2 dogs. DC effectively recovered heartbeats under Impella support in one dog but not in any dog under ECMO support. (*From* [*A*] Tuseth V, Pettersen RJ, Grong K, et al. Randomised comparison of percutaneous left ventricular assist device with open-chest cardiac massage and with surgical assist device during ischaemic cardiac arrest. Resuscitation 2010;81(11):1566–70; with permission; [*B*] Kawashima D, Gojo S, Nishimura T, et al. Left ventricular mechanical support with Impella provides more ventricular unloading in heart failure than extracorporeal membrane oxygenation. ASAIO J 2011;57(3):169–76; with permission.)

PVAD in Experimental Cardiac Arrest

Specific assessment of the effect of a percutaneous device during cardiac arrest has been performed in recently published experimental protocols on swine. The experimental findings show the potential of a continuous-flow PVAD to sustain circulation during cardiac arrest and indicate a possible clinical usefulness of such devices. Intravenous fluid loading seems to improve clinical efficacy. Available data indicate that a percutaneous intracardiac impeller device may be able to sustain both myocardial and cerebral perfusion at a clinically relevant level during persistent ischemic cardiac arrest. Myocardial and cerebral blood flow could be maintained during prolonged VF.

Furthermore, the assessment of metabolic markers in the brain during VF using intracerebral microdialysis indicates ischemic brain injury may be avoided during 20 to 40 minutes of cardiac arrest without simultaneous chest compressions.[32]

In another study, the Impella 2.5 achieved hemodynamics and ROSC after defibrillation comparable with optimal conventional resuscitation with open-chest manual cardiac massage (OCCM) during 20 minutes of VF (**Fig. 7**).[55]

THERAPEUTIC OPTIONS

PVAD support represents a future potential for improving outcomes in patients with acute cardiac collapse and critical cerebral hypoperfusion secondary to acute heart failure or cardiac arrest. The use of Impella support during coronary revascularization in cardiac arrest can be of particular advantage because revascularization could be performed without concomitant chest compressions and without the use vasopressor drugs. If spontaneous circulation is restored, the unloading effect of a PVAD should be beneficial for myocardial oxygen consumption and recovery. Improved vital organ perfusion can further improve prognosis. The use of PVAD therapy in patients with cardiac arrest may be relevant as an adjunct to established resuscitation with chest compressions with a possible synergistic effect on vital organ blood delivery. Further benefit of PVAD therapy may be possible with a device that is able to obviate chest compressions and vasopressor during VF, allowing for optimal coronary revascularization and medical stabilization of patients. To achieve this, blood delivery from the device should be sufficient to prevent acute cerebral injury. The general hemodynamic and clinical effects of the device should not be inferior to established methods for CPR. In some cases, the use of impeller support with concomitant CPR or even with ECMO could be desirable to achieve optimal circulation and unloading.

Impella

Hemodynamic support in cardiac arrest should sustain sufficient vital organ perfusion to avoid ischemic injury to allow for the treatment of the underlying disease. Moreover, the intervention should be readily available, easy to establish, and any risk of complications should be minimized. PVAD therapy, in particular using rapidly deployed Impella devices, has the potential to fulfill these criteria (**Box 3**).

Technical Advantages

The generally smaller size and, thus, minimal vascular trauma with percutaneous devices can reduce the risk of bleeding and vascular compromise during implantation and use. By permitting rapid hemodynamic support with less complicated implantation procedures, a percutaneous approach seems especially useful for patients with acute circulatory collapse. In cardiac arrest, the compromise between sizes versus output of such devices may be outweighed by the easy and rapid deployment of the smaller devices.

LP 2.5

The Impella 2.5 is a miniature impeller pump placed retrograde into the left ventricle via a 13F femoral artery sheath. The impeller pump has capacity to pump 2.5 L of blood per minute into the ascending aorta in the level of the coronary artery ostia. Placement into the left ventricle is rapid, and the risk of complications is low. In severe shock, the potential of the Impella 2.5 for improving blood flow to the heart and brain has been indicated in clinical studies. Also, systemic blood delivery may be sufficient to prevent short-term tissue ischemia. In resuscitated patients, myocardial and cerebral hypoperfusion are major contributing factors for clinical outcomes in survivors. The Impella has its outlet proximal to the coronary and carotid arteries in the ascending aorta, which allows for preferential flow to the cerebral and myocardial vessels. The use of PVADs may have the potential to prevent ischemic damage to the heart and brain and improve clinical outcomes for cardiac arrest survivors.

Unloading

The intracardiac impeller device also has potential to reduce left ventricular pressures by delivering blood into the systemic circulation. During cardiac arrest, left ventricular unloading can immediately improve the chances for successful ROSC both by relieving ischemia and by reducing intracardiac pressure. Unloading may also be of benefit during reperfusion and recovery.

PVAD in Resuscitation

Even with successful optimal treatment and ROSC, cerebral injury is still a problem in patients surviving the acute phase after cardiac arrest. The hemodynamic efficacy of chest compressions is often limited, unpredictable, and cannot be maintained over time. PVAD support may have the potential to significantly improve results by augmenting the delivery of oxygenated blood to vital organs during resuscitation.

Blood Delivery

With a PVAD in place, the delivery of oxygenated blood to the arterial circulation depends on

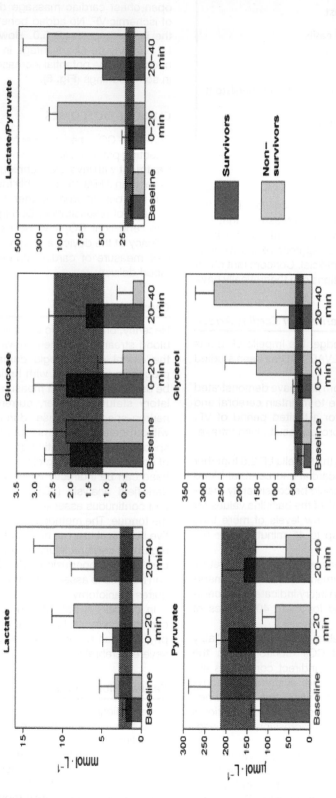

Fig. 7. Cerebral microdialysis during prolonged VF with Impella support. (*From* Tuseth V, Pettersen RJ, Epstein A, et al. Percutaneous left ventricular assist device can prevent acute cerebral ischaemia during ventricular fibrillation. Resuscitation 2009;80(10):1197–203; with permission.)

Box 3
Impella in cardiac arrest

- Deploys rapidly and easily
- Unloads the left ventricle
- Provides vital organ perfusion
- Promising experimental data in persistent arrest
- Small and large devices used
- Useful in AMI with persistent arrest?

---

adequate filling of the left heart from the pulmonary circulation. In resuscitation, blood flow from the right to left heart is limited. Measures that improve venous return can augment the available left-side blood volumes. Aggressive intravenous fluid loading may be beneficial. Concomitant chest or abdominal compressions can theoretically have a positive effect.

Experience From Experimental Cardiac Arrest

To the author's knowledge, the Impella LP 2.5 is the only percutaneous LVAD that has been studied during cardiac arrest.

Experimental data from pigs have demonstrated the ability of this device to maintain cerebral and myocardial perfusion for a limited period of VF. One study showed improved results with intravenous fluid loading.

In one protocol using the Impella LP 2.5 together with fluid loading, myocardial and cerebral blood flow by microspheres could be consistently maintained at more than 60% of the baseline values for a limited period. Blood flow levels of more than 40% were sustained up to 45 minutes after the onset of VF.[32]

Cerebral ischemia was assessed with cerebral microdialysis. Measurements of metabolic markers of hypoxia and brain injury indicated that cerebral injury was avoided for 20 to 40 minutes of cardiac arrest.

Brain injury and cerebral perfusion was reliably indicated by end-tidal CO_2 monitoring via the ventilator, which allowed indirect continuous assessment of cerebral and systemic hemodynamics. Moreover, data were favorable when compared with the previous data for conventional resuscitation with chest compressions and vasopressor therapy.[54]

The most recent study compared the Impella LP 2.5 with optimal conventional manual resuscitation with open-chest cardiac massage and with a larger LVAD (LP 5.0). With the Impella LP 2.5, cerebral perfusion, hemodynamics, and rates of successful defibrillation were as good as with the open-chest cardiac massage during 15 minutes of ischemic VF. No added benefit was found with the larger Impella LP 5.0. However, the Impella LP 5.0 may be of advantage in selected patients because of the potential increase in blood delivery in some settings (**Fig. 8**).

CLINICAL OUTCOMES

End-tidal CO_2 measurements may be useful in selecting patients with survival potential for further treatment with invasive techniques (**Box 4**). Values lower than 2 kPa can possibly identify patients that will not benefit from further treatment after 20 minutes of resuscitation. During mechanical support, end-tidal CO_2 can be used to assess the efficacy of the device and can be used as an indirect measure of cardiac output and vital organ blood delivery.

Cerebral Monitoring

Recently, brain-specific peptides released into the blood stream have been shown to correlate with the extent of neurologic damage and with the prognosis for patients with brain injury and could be useful as an indirect measure of cerebral circulatory status. However, current data assessing neuron-specific enolase during LVAD support without cerebral ischemia found results to be unspecific and interpretation unclear in the presence of concomitant cardiac disease. Blood flow to the head can be indirectly assessed with sidestream dark-field analysis (SDF), which permits direct and continuous assessment of microcirculation in the tongue. The method is easy to use and attractive in clinical use but has not been validated with regard to cerebral injury or neurologic injury after cerebral hypoperfusion. Cerebral microdialysis can be used to assess cerebral metabolism but requires craniotomy.

In critically ill patients on sedation, electroencephalography and cerebral computed tomography (CT) can be used to assess the likelihood of severe cerebral injury.

Cardiac Monitoring

Echocardiography should be routinely performed to assess left and right heart functional status and filling.

Additional monitoring with invasive Swan-Ganz, measurements can be helpful in optimizing adjunctive treatment. After the initial critical phase, noninvasive hemodynamic monitoring can be sufficient in stabilized patients.

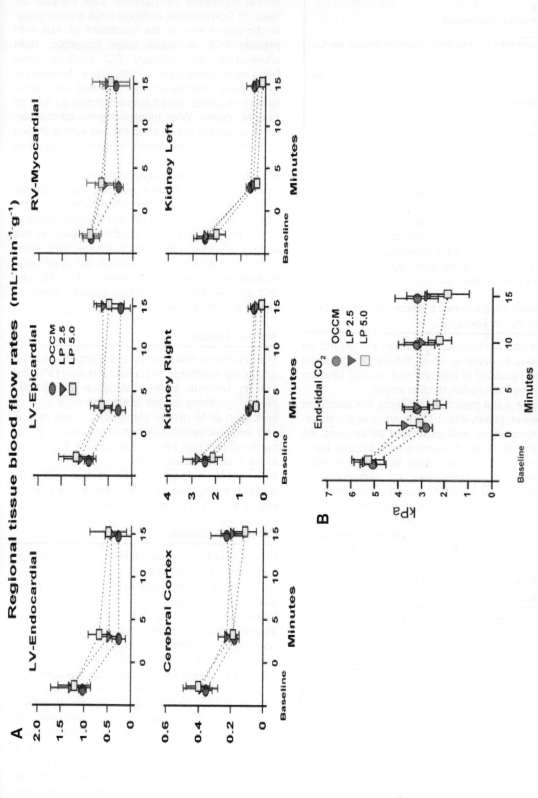

Fig. 8. (A) Blood flow with microspheres to vital organs during cardiac arrest with Impella support. (B) End-tidal CO_2 during cardiac arrest with Impella support. (*From* Tuseth V, Pettersen RJ, Grong K, et al. Randomised comparison of percutaneous left ventricular assist device with open-chest cardiac massage and with surgical assist device during ischaemic cardiac arrest. Resuscitation 2010;81(11):1566–70; with permission.)

Box 4
Monitoring treatment

- End-tidal CO_2 can indicate vital organ perfusion during arrest.
- Cerebral monitoring with blood flow and metabolic assessment is possible in comatose patients.
- Use echocardiography for assessing cardiac function.

Hemodynamics

Intra-arterial and intravenous pressure monitoring according to routine practice is feasible during PCI with LVAD support during cardiac arrest. SDF, Near Infrared Spectrophotometry, and peripheral transcutaneous oximetry may add further relevant information.

Cessation of Treatment, Recovery, or Heart Replacement Therapy

Mechanical hemodynamic support should not be continued in patients when definite clinical signs of initial recovery of cerebral and cardiac function cannot be found after cardiac arrest.

If, after initial treatment, patients are stabilized and neurologically intact, hemodynamic and echocardiographic as well as clinical parameters are used to determine if weaning from Impella treatment can be performed (**Box 5**). In patients who are unable to sustain adequate hemodynamics without Impella support, more permanent heart replacement therapy with surgical LVAD or heart transplantation should be considered. This process of possible outcomes evaluation should be initiated early in the PVAD treatment period.

COMPLICATIONS AND CONCERNS
Logistic Challenges

Implementation of prehospital and in-hospital logistics (chain of life) is critical for optimal results

---

Box 5
Treatment follow-up

- Complications rare
- Close monitoring required
- Continuous assessment of prognosis
  - Stop treatment
  - Wean
  - Continue as bridge therapy

---

in the treatment of patients with cardiac arrest.[1,55] Comparable routines have shown prognostic effect also in the treatment of AMI with primary PCI. In most large hospitals, both chain-of-life and primary PCI routines have been established over several years. Adequately functioning routines are documented with satisfactory response and treatment times as well as clinical results. With most ischemic cardiac arrests occurring out of hospital and with a limited time window for life-saving intervention, decision making and transport must be organized in a structured, efficient algorithm. The use of a mechanical CPR device may be useful during transportation. A catheterization laboratory with trained personnel must be alerted and ready at arrival to the hospital for eligible patients. In this setting, it necessary with a cooperative effort involving EMS and acute cardiac catheterization facilities to achieve the potential of PVAD and PCI intervention in persistent cardiac arrest to show clinical benefit.

Technical Issues

The placement and function of the Impella must be cautiously monitored, in particular during CPR and moving patients when dislocation can occur. Alarm algorithms on the device console give an indication as to proper placement, pump output, and also mechanical function of the device. Echocardiography can be used to assess the proper location of the device in the LV and aorta. In addition, chest radiographs should be performed routinely during use for supplementary information with regard to optimal deployment.

Cerebral Perfusion

Severe neurologic impairment is not common during long-term LVAD use.

As for cardiopulmonary bypass, cerebral blood flow and cerebral perfusion pressure is likely related to device output. According to currently available data, no cerebral embolic complications have been reported with the PVAD devices. However, only limited patient data have been published; the specific assessment of cerebral injury has, to the author's knowledge, not been assessed during clinical PVAD support. In experimental cardiac arrest, cerebral perfusion and metabolism was maintained at sufficient levels for a limited time. Vasopressor therapy, inotropes, and blood transfusions may be useful in preventing cerebral ischemia during controlled cardioplegia and in heart failure but may be counterproductive in the treatment of acute circulatory collapse.

Embolization

Intra-arterial device therapy can theoretically be complicated by the introduction of air and thrombi, which may embolize into the cerebral circulation and contribute to brain injury. The devices may further cause blood clot activation and thrombus dislodgement because of blood flow turbulence from the pumps. Also, mechanical fragmentation of aortic plaque material and leakage of air via the intravascular catheters can occur during use. With current surgical heart assist technologies and adequate anticoagulation, the risk of clinically relevant embolization has been minimized. It is likely that with cautious implantation and adequate anticoagulation, the risk of cerebral damage caused by PVAD systems may be comparable with conventional cardiac catheterization procedures.

Output Limitations

Although initial experimental findings suggest that percutaneous LVAD support sustains vital organ perfusion during cardiac arrest, previous studies have indicated only limited clinical effect of LVAD support despite initially promising hemodynamic data. Current experimental data from PVAD support during VF should obviously be interpreted with caution based on these previous experiences.

In clinical use, the larger Impella LP 5.0 of similar design with maximum output of 5 L per minute is often preferred to the smaller LP 2.5 because of the higher delivery and increased mechanical stability. The LP 5.0 is more bulky and requires surgical cut down for arterial access; thus, implantation can be somewhat more complicated than for the true percutaneous version. Once inserted, the larger device can achieve higher systemic blood delivery and could have the potential to improve hemodynamics compared with the LP 2.5. However, the device requires sufficient filling from the right side to achieve its output potential, and efficacy may be limited by poor filling of the left ventricle. Experimental data indicate this may be a particular issue during VF when sufficient circulating blood volumes can rarely be obtained. Possibly, the presence of aortic regurgitation may limit the efficacy of the larger devices in this particular setting. Interestingly, a new Impella device with 14F size and 4-L delivery is currently in limited clinical use but is not freely available yet.

Complications

Very few complications have been reported during clinical use and deployment of Impella devices. Transient hemolysis is routinely noted but not considered a clinical problem.

Possible device-related serious complications are mainly mechanical or related to the risk of thromboembolism and bleeding. Although rare, such complications may be critical and include access site bleeding, ischemic lower limb complications, stroke, and also aortic valvulopathy.

SUMMARY

Persistent cardiac arrest is often caused by coronary ischemia. Urgent revascularization during on-going resuscitation with PVAD support may be feasible and can have the potential to improve the prognosis.

Transport during resuscitation is a challenge that may be overcome with the use of CPR devices. In the catheterization laboratory, rapid deployment of PVAD may reduce ischemia and contribute to electrical stabilization of the heart as well as facilitate definite treatment with PCI. After revascularization, PVAD therapy may promote myocardial recovery and improve vital organ perfusion in a critical phase.

Based on limited existing evidence, the use of PCI and Impella support in selected cases of refractory cardiac arrest may be considered. This field should be further investigated with structured randomized trials for conclusive results.

REFERENCES

1. Nolan JP, Soar J, Zideman DA, et al, On behalf of the ERC Guidelines Writing Group. European Resuscitation Council Guidelines for Resuscitation 2010. Resuscitation 2010;81(10):1219–451.
2. Silfvast T. Cause of death in unsuccessful prehospital resuscitation. J Intern Med 1991;229:331–5.
3. Zheng ZJ, Croft JB, Giles WH, et al. Sudden cardiac death in the United States, 1989 to 1998. Circulation 2001;104:2158–63.
4. Atwood C, Eisenberg MS, Herlitz J, et al. Incidence of EMS-treated out-of-hospital cardiac arrest in Europe. Resuscitation 2005;67:75–80.
5. Kummen L, Holager BK, Heltne JK. Hjertestans i Bergensområdet. Student særemne, Norway: University of Bergen; 2010.
6. Nichol G, Thomas E, Callaway CW, et al. Regional variation in out-of-hospital cardiac arrest incidence and outcome. JAMA 2008;300:1423–31.
7. Iwami T, Nichol G, Hiraide A, et al. Continuous improvements in "chain of survival" increased survival after out-of-hospital cardiac arrests: a large-scale population-based study. Circulation 2009; 119:728–34.

8. Layon AJ, Gabrielli A, Goldfeder BW, et al. Utstein style analysis of rural out-of-hospital cardiac arrest [OOHCA]: total cardiopulmonary resuscitation (CPR) time inversely correlates with hospital discharge rate. Resuscitation 2003;56:59–66.

9. Sunde K, Pytte M, Jacobsen D, et al. Implementation of a standardised treatment protocol for post resuscitation care after out-of-hospital cardiac arrest. Resuscitation 2007;73:29–39.

10. Ewy GA, Kern KB. Recent advances in cardiopulmonary resuscitation: cardiocerebral resuscitation. J Am Coll Cardiol 2009;53:149–57.

11. Meaney PA, Nadkarni VM, Kern KB, et al. Rhythms and outcomes of adult in-hospital cardiac arrest. Crit Care Med 2010;38:101–8.

12. Eftestol T, Wik L, Sunde K, et al. Effects of cardiopulmonary resuscitation on predictors of ventricular fibrillation defibrillation success during out-of-hospital cardiac arrest. Circulation 2004;110:10–5.

13. Hallstrom AP, Ornato JP, Weisfeldt M, et al, Public Access Defibrillation Trial Investigators. Public-access defibrillation and survival after out-of-hospital cardiac arrest. N Engl J Med 2004; 351:637–46.

14. Spaulding CM, Joly LM, Rosenberg A, et al. Immediate coronary angiography in survivors of out-of-hospital cardiac arrest. N Engl J Med 1997;336: 1629–33.

15. Lowel H, Meisinger C, Heier M, et al. Sex specific trends of sudden cardiac death and acute myocardial infarction: results of the population-based KORA/MONICA-Augsburg register 1985 to 1998. Dtsch Med Wochenschr 2002;127:2311–6.

16. Quintero-Moran B, Moreno R, Villarreal S, et al. Percutaneous coronary intervention for cardiac arrest secondary to ST-elevation acute myocardial infarction. Influence of immediate paramedical/medical assistance on clinical outcome. J Invasive Cardiol 2006;18:269–72.

17. Herlitz J, Ekstrom L, Axelsson A, et al. Continuation of CPR on admission to emergency department after out-of-hospital cardiac arrest. Occurrence, characteristics and outcome. Resuscitation 1997; 33:223–31.

18. Dorian P, Cass D, Schwartz B, et al. Amiodarone as compared with lidocaine for shock-resistant ventricular fibrillation. N Engl J Med 2002;346:884–90.

19. Nielsen N, Sandhall L, Schersten F, et al. Successful resuscitation with mechanical CPR, therapeutic hypothermia and coronary intervention during manual CPR after out-of-hospital cardiac arrest. Resuscitation 2005;65:111–3.

20. Larsen AI, Hjørnevik A, Bonarjee V, et al. Coronary blood flow and perfusion pressure during coronary angiography in patients with ongoing mechanical chest compression: a report on 6 cases. Resuscitation 2010;81(4):493–7.

21. Niemann JT, Rosborough JP, Youngquist S, et al. Is all ventricular fibrillation the same? A comparison of ischemically induced with electrically induced ventricular fibrillation in a porcine cardiac arrest and resuscitation model. Crit Care Med 2007;35: 1356–61.

22. Ristagno G, Tang W, Xu TY, et al. Outcomes of CPR in the presence of partial occlusion of left anterior descending coronary artery. Resuscitation 2007; 75:357–65.

23. Ono H, Osanai T, Ishizaka H, et al. Nicorandil improves cardiac function and clinical outcome in patients with acute myocardial infarction undergoing primary percutaneous coronary intervention: role of inhibitory effect on reactive oxygen species formation. Am Heart J 2004;148(4):E15.

24. Gomez L, Li B, Mewton N, et al. Inhibition of mitochondrial permeability transition pore opening: translation to patients. Cardiovasc Res 2009; 83(2):226–33.

25. Indik JH, Allen D, Shanmugasundaram M, et al. Predictors of resuscitation in a swine model of ischemic and nonischemic ventricular fibrillation cardiac arrest: superiority of amplitude spectral area and slope to predict a return of spontaneous circulation when resuscitation efforts are prolonged. Crit Care Med 2010;38(12):2352–7.

26. Tukkie R, Gründeman PF, Moulijn AC, et al. Treatment of intractable ventricular fibrillation with prompt circulatory support using a biventricular assist device in pigs–an experimental study. Thorac Cardiovasc Surg 1992;40(1):5–9.

27. Falk JL, Rackow EC, Weil MH. End-tidal carbondioxide concentration during cardiopulmonary resuscitation. N Engl J Med 1988;318:607–11.

28. Gudipati CV, Weil MH, Bisera J, et al. Expired carbon dioxide: a noninvasive monitor of cardiopulmonary resuscitation. Circulation 1988;77:234–9.

29. Weil MH, Bisera J, Trevino RP, et al. Cardiac output and end-tidal carbon dioxide. Crit Care Med 1985; 13:907–9.

30. Gazmuri RJ, Kube E. Capnography during cardiac resuscitation: a clue on mechanisms and a guide to interventions. Crit Care Med 2003;7:411–2.

31. Wayne MA, Levine RL, Miller CC. Use of end-tidal carbon dioxide to predict outcome in prehospital cardiac arrest. N Engl J Med 1997;337:301–6.

32. Tuseth V, Pettersen RJ, Epstein A, et al. Percutaneous left ventricular assist device can prevent acute cerebral ischaemia during ventricular fibrillation. Resuscitation 2009;80(10):1197–203.

33. Müller S, How OJ, Hermansen SE, et al. Vasopressin impairs brain, heart and kidney perfusion: an experimental study in pigs after transient myocardial ischemia. Crit Care 2008;12:R20.

34. Gedeborg R, Silander HC, Rubertsson S, et al. Cerebral ischaemia in experimental cardiopulmonary

resuscitation—comparison of epinephrine and aortic occlusion. Resuscitation 2001;50:319–29.

35. Olasveengen TM, Sunde K, Brunborg C, et al. Intravenous drug administration during out-of-hospital cardiac arrest: a randomized trial. JAMA 2009;302:2222–9.

36. Ristagno G, Tang W, Huang L, et al. Epinephrine reduces cerebral perfusion during cardiopulmonary resuscitation. Crit Care Med 2009;37(4):1408–15.

37. Lindner KH, Pfenninger EG, Lurie KG, et al. Effects of active compression-decompression resuscitation on myocardial and cerebral blood flow in pigs. Circulation 1993;88:1254–63.

38. Halperin HR, Paradis N, Ornato JP, et al. Cardiopulmonary resuscitation with a novel chest compression device in a porcine model of cardiac arrest: improved hemodynamics and mechanisms. J Am Coll Cardiol 2004;44:2214–20.

39. Steen S, Liao Q, Pierre L, et al. Evaluation of LUCAS, a new device for automatic mechanical compression and active decompression resuscitation. Resuscitation 2002;55:285–99.

40. Rubertsson S, Karlsten R. Increased cortical cerebral blood flow with LUCAS; a new device for mechanical chest compressions compared to standard external compressions during experimental cardiopulmonary resuscitation. Resuscitation 2005;65:357–63.

41. Chen JM, DeRose JJ, Slater JP, et al. Improved survival rates support left ventricular assist device implantation early after myocardial infarction. J Am Coll Cardiol 1999;33:1903–8.

42. Wohlschlaeger J, Meier B, Schmitz KJ, et al. Cardiomyocyte survivin protein expression is associated with cell size and DNA content in the failing human heart and is reversibly regulated after ventricular unloading. J Heart Lung Transplant 2010;29(11):1286–92.

43. Son HS, Sun K, Fang YH, et al. The effects of pulsatile versus non-pulsatile extracorporeal circulation on the pattern of coronary artery blood flow during cardiac arrest. Int J Artif Organs 2005;28:609–16.

44. Feller ED, Sorensen EN, Haddad M, et al. Clinical outcomes are similar in pulsatile and nonpulsatile left ventricular assist device recipients. Ann Thorac Surg 2007;83:1082–8.

45. Dang NC, Topkara VK, Leacche M, et al. Left ventricular assist device implantation after acute anterior wall myocardial infarction and cardiogenic shock: a two-center study. J Thorac Cardiovasc Surg 2005;130:693–8.

46. Miller LW, Pagani FD, Russell SD, et al, HeartMate II Clinical Investigators. Use of a continuous-flow device in patients awaiting heart transplantation. N Engl J Med 2007;357:885–96.

47. Massetti M, Tasle M, Le Page O, et al. Back from irreversibility: extracorporeal life support for prolonged cardiac arrest. Ann Thorac Surg 2005;79:178–83.

48. Martin GB, Rivers EP, Paradis NA, et al. Emergency department cardiopulmonary bypass in the treatment of human cardiac arrest. Chest 1998;113:743–51.

49. Shin JS, Lee SW, Han GS, et al. Successful extracorporeal life support in cardiac arrest with recurrent ventricular fibrillation unresponsive to standard cardiopulmonary resuscitation. Resuscitation 2007;73:309–13.

50. Henriques JP, Remmelink M, Baan J Jr, et al. Safety and feasibility of elective high-risk percutaneous coronary intervention procedures with left ventricular support of the Impella Recover LP 2.5. Am J Cardiol 2006;97:990–2.

51. Tang GHL, Malekan M, Kai M, et al. Peripheral venoarterial extracorporeal membrane oxygenation improves survival in myocardial infarction with cardiogenic shock. J Thorac Cardiovasc Surg 2013;145(3):e32–3.

52. Valgimigli M, Steendijk P, Sianos G, et al. Left ventricular unloading and concomitant total cardiac output increase by the use of percutaneous Impella Recover LP 2.5 assist device during high-risk coronary intervention. Catheter Cardiovasc Interv 2005;65:263–7.

53. Seyfarth M, Sibbing D, Bauer I, et al. A randomized clinical trial to evaluate the safety and efficacy of a percutaneous left ventricular assist device versus intra-aortic balloon pumping for treatment of cardiogenic shock caused by myocardial infarction. J Am Coll Cardiol 2008;52:1584–8.

54. Patanè F, Zingarelli E, Sansone F, et al. Acute ventricular septal defect treated with an Impella recovery as a 'bridge therapy' to heart transplantation. Interact Cardiovasc Thorac Surg 2007;6(6):818–9.

55. Tuseth V, Pettersen RJ, Grong K, et al. Randomised comparison of percutaneous left ventricular assist device with open-chest cardiac massage and with surgical assist device during ischaemic cardiac arrest. Resuscitation 2010;81(11):1566–70.

Percutaneous Circulatory Assist Devices for Right Ventricular Failure

Navin K. Kapur, MD[a],*, Yousef H. Bader, MD[b]

KEYWORDS

- Ventricular assist device • Right ventricle • Cardiogenic shock • Heart failure

KEY POINTS

- Right ventricular (RV) failure is a major determinant of clinical outcomes in patients with acute myocardial infarction, left heart failure, and pulmonary hypertension and after cardiac surgery.
- Anatomic and physiologic determinants of RV function are distinct from the left ventricle; therefore, management of RV failure and cardiogenic shock must be tailored accordingly.
- Percutaneous circulatory support devices for RV failure are relatively new with limited clinical data examining their utility; however, the potential beneficial impact of these devices will likely be determined by optimal patient-device matching, timing of device deployment, and the development of optimal weaning algorithms.

 Videos of a right ventricular assist device implantation accompany this article at http://www.interventional.theclinics.com/

INTRODUCTION

Heart failure is a major cause of global morbidity and mortality affecting nearly 24 million individuals worldwide. An estimated 2.6% of the US population suffers from congestive heart failure, with an additional 500,000 new cases diagnosed each year.[1] Although most clinical and preclinical science has focused on left ventricular (LV) failure, the importance of right ventricular (RV) function has become more apparent over the past few decades. Causes of RV failure can be broadly categorized into 3 groups: (1) direct RV myocyte injury in the setting of myocardial infarction (MI), myocarditis, or after cardiac surgery; (2) volume overload secondary to right-sided valvular insufficiency or after placement of an LV assist device (LVAD); and (3) pressure overload caused by pulmonary hypertension, pulmonic valve stenosis, or a pulmonary embolus. Regardless of the mechanism, the presence of RV dysfunction is a primary determinant of functional capacity and prognosis. In the setting of LV failure, acute MI (AMI), chronic lung disease, pulmonary hypertension, congenital heart disease, or acute pulmonary embolus, concomitant RV dysfunction is associated with higher morbidity and short-term mortality.[2–9]

The most common cause of RV failure is LV failure is a mantra that has been repeated for decades and is based on the concept that

Funding Sources: None.

Conflicts of Interest: Preclinical research support from Heartware Inc and CardiacAssist Inc. Speaker honoraria/consultant: Maquet Inc and Thoratec Inc (N.K. Kapur); none (Y.H. Bader).

[a] The Cardiovascular Center, Tufts Medical Center, 800 Washington Street, Box #80, Boston, MA 02111, USA;
[b] Department of Cardiology, The Cardiovascular Center, Tufts Medical Center, 800 Washington Street, Boston, MA 02111, USA
* Corresponding author.
E-mail address: nkapur@tuftsmedicalcenter.org

Intervent Cardiol Clin 2 (2013) 445–456
http://dx.doi.org/10.1016/j.iccl.2013.04.001
2211-7458/13/$ – see front matter © 2013 Published by Elsevier Inc.

chronically elevated pulmonary venous pressures associated with LV failure promote adverse RV remodeling. However, few studies have examined the impact of pulmonary venous hypertension (PVH) in the setting of left ventricular failure on RV structure and function. Recent estimates indicate that nearly 70% of individuals with heart failure on the left side of the heart have PVH, yet the fundamental mechanisms underlying the development of RV dysfunction in left-side heart failure remain poorly understood.[10] Several studies have shown that the presence of elevated pulmonary artery systolic pressure in patients with heart failure on the left side of the heart was inversely associated with RV ejection fraction and directly associated with increased mortality.[11]

Over the past 6 decades, therapeutic options for patients with end-stage left-side heart failure have grown rapidly. Cardiac transplantation has become more feasible with improved long-term outcomes because of advances in immunosuppressive regimens and myocardial preservation techniques.[12] Surgically implanted LVADs have also evolved from large, extracorporeal pulsatile systems to smaller, fully implantable continuous-flow devices that are associated with improved long-term morbidity and mortality. However, despite advances in left-sided therapeutic options, the presence of RV dysfunction remains a major cause of mortality after heart transplantation and LVAD placement. Among heart transplant recipients, 2% to 3% of patients will develop some degree of RV dysfunction in the perioperative setting, which is associated with a 4- to 5-fold increase in short-term mortality.[13] Among LVAD recipients, the incidence of RV failure ranges from 5% to 44% and depends on the criteria used to define RV failure. Among patients with RV failure after LVAD placement, an RV support device was required in 16% to 100% of patients and in-hospital mortality ranged between 24% and 83%.[14] These findings highlight the importance of RV failure in the advanced heart failure population.

Several studies have examined the clinical importance of RV failure in the setting of an AMI. RV dysfunction as defined by echocardiography can be identified in up to 50% of patients presenting with an acute Inferior Wall Myocardial Infarction (IWMI).[15–17] Of these patients, 15% to 25% will exhibit hemodynamic instability suggestive of RV involvement, yet histologic infarction of the RV free wall occurs in only 3% to 5% of patients with an acute IWMI.[18] In a substudy of the Should We Emergently Revascularize Occluded Coronaries for Cardiogenic Shock (SHOCK) trial, RV-dominant cardiogenic shock was associated with similar in-hospital mortality rates as LV-dominant cardiogenic shock (53.1% vs 60.8%, $P = .3$) despite a younger age, lower rate of anterior MI, and higher likelihood of single-vessel disease among patients with RV-dominant shock.[4] Furthermore, a meta-analysis of several studies showed significantly higher in-hospital mortality and a higher incidence of shock, ventricular arrhythmias, and advanced atrioventricular block if AMI involved the RV.[19]

Contemporary management of RV failure includes reversal of the primary cause, volume resuscitation, inotropic support, and pulmonary vasodilation, which serve to maintain RV preload, enhance RV contractility, and reduce RV afterload, respectively.[20] In refractory RV failure, treatment options are limited to surgical RV assist devices (RVAD), extracorporeal membrane oxygenation (ECMO), atrial septostomy, and cardiac transplantation. Percutaneously delivered circulatory support for RV failure is an emerging field with several device options available, including the intra-aortic balloon pump (IABP), the Tandem-Heart (CardiacAssist Inc, Pittsburgh, PA) centrifugal flow pump, the axial-flow Impella RP catheter (Abiomed Inc, Danvers, MA), and the veno-arterial ECMO (VA-ECMO).[21] Appropriate patient-device selection, timing of device use, weaning parameters, and the hemodynamic impact of each device remains poorly understood and represents a new era in percutaneous therapies for patients with advanced heart failure.

RV ANATOMY AND PHYSIOLOGY

Several developmental and anatomic features distinguish the RV from the LV. During embryonic development, the RV and RV outflow tract originate from cells of the anterior (secondary) heart field, whereas the LV and atria originate from the primary heart field.[22] Anatomically, the RV free wall is thin (2–3 mm), compliant, and forms a hemi-ellipsoid shape that adheres to the LV. A large sinus for venous inflow and a tubular outflow tract provide a funnel-like configuration to the heavily trabeculated RV. Unlike the shared annulus of the aortic and mitral valves, the crista supraventricularis is a unique muscle bridge that separates the RV inflow (tricuspid annulus) from the outflow tract (pulmonic annulus). Normal RV function is also distinct from the LV and is governed by pulmonary vascular resistance, systemic venous return, pericardial compliance, and native contractility of both the RV free wall and interventricular septum.[23] As compared with LV function, generating RV output requires one-sixth the energy expenditure because most of the RV stroke work maintains forward momentum of blood flow into a highly compliant, low-resistance pulmonic circulation.[24] In the pressure-volume domain, this environment results in a hemodynamic signature unique to the RV that lacks isovolumic phases of contraction and relaxation throughout systole and diastole. In the setting of acute right coronary artery (RCA) occlusion, prior studies in large animal models have shown that RV ischemia causes the pressure volume loop to shift toward increased RV volume, decreased RV pressure, reduced RV stroke volume, and increased RV wall stress (**Fig. 1**).[25]

Afterload is a major determinant of RV function. For this reason, several additional hemodynamic variables should be considered when examining the hemodynamics of RV function. First, ventriculo-arterial coupling describes the impact of arterial loading conditions on ventricular function. Under any given condition, optimal pump efficiency is achieved if ventricular function, or end-systolic elastance, is matched by vascular load, also known as arterial elastance.[26–28] The RV is exquisitely sensitive to increased afterload such that minor increments cause dramatic reductions in RV stroke volume. Second, ventriculo-ventricular coupling

refers to the influence one ventricle has on the other.[29,30] Under conditions of pressure and volume overload within an intact pericardium, reduced RV output decreases LV preload and mechanically impedes LV diastole, thereby reducing the net LV stroke volume. RV overload also limits LV coronary blood flow by reducing LV output and elevating coronary sinus pressure.[31–33] The impact of progressive LV failure on RV function remains poorly understood. Third, RV afterload itself is determined by 3 primary factors, namely, pulmonary vascular resistance (PVR), pulmonary vascular compliance (PVC), and pulmonary vascular impedance (PVI).[34–36] Recent studies have shown that increased filling pressures on the left side of the heart serve as an amplifier that enhances vascular impedance and results in increased RV afterload.[37] Thus, all 3 components of RV afterload are influenced by acute (PVI) and chronic (PVC and PVR) increases in filling pressures on the left side of the heart.

The clinical pathophysiology of RV failure depends on the primary cause. Acute RV failure can occur in the setting of ischemia, caused by either a coronary occlusion or after open heart surgery, and can occur after direct myocyte injury secondary to myocarditis. In these settings, RV failure is characterized by both RV systolic and biventricular diastolic failure (**Fig. 2**). More commonly after acute proximal RCA occlusion, both RV free wall and interventricular septal ischemia reduce RV cardiac output and a subsequent reduction in LV preload.[38] RV ischemia also impairs RV diastolic function, which in combination with RV systolic failure causes RV pressure and volume overload with subsequent RV dilation.[39] After LVAD implantation, increased venous return to the RV can cause volume overload and lead to RV dilatation.[40] In the setting of primary or secondary pulmonary hypertension, increased RV afterload leads to RV hypertrophy and fibrosis, which ultimately contributes to adverse cardiac remodeling and progressive RV failure. Regardless of the primary cause of RV failure, in the presence of an intact pericardium, RV dilation compresses the LV cavity, thereby equalizing biventricular diastolic filling pressures. The combination of RV systolic and biventricular diastolic dysfunction reduces systemic cardiac output, worsens renal and hepatic congestion, and impairs global coronary blood flow.

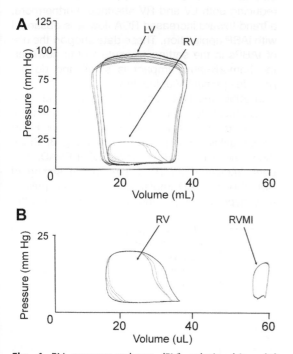

Fig. 1. RV pressure-volume (PV) relationships. (*A*) Normal LV and RV PV loops showing differences in the magnitude of pressure and contrasting the isovolumic phases of LV contraction compared with nonisovolumic contraction in the RV. (*B*) Changes in the RV PV relationship induced by acute RVMI. RV volume is increased, whereas RV pressure and stroke volume (width of the PV loop) are reduced.

CIRCULATORY SUPPORT DEVICES FOR RV FAILURE

Over the past 3 decades, mechanical support devices for right-side heart failure have passed through several generations of development.

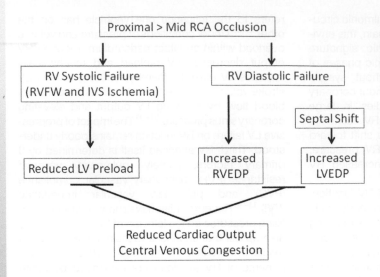

Fig. 2. Pathophysiology of RV failure. More commonly after acute proximal RCA occlusion, both RV free-wall (RVFW) and interventricular septal (IVS) ischemia reduce RV cardiac output and a subsequent reduction in LV preload. RV ischemia also impairs RV diastolic function, which in combination with RV systolic failure causes RV pressure and volume overload with subsequent RV dilation. In the presence of an intact pericardium, RV dilation compresses the LV cavity, thereby increasing and equalizing biventricular diastolic filling pressures. The combination of RV systolic and biventricular diastolic dysfunction reduces systemic cardiac output, worsens renal and hepatic congestion, and impairs global coronary blood flow. RVEDP, Right ventricular end diastolic pressure.

First-generation, surgically implanted RV pumps were pulsatile with valves located within the inflow and outflow segments.[41] Early attempts at dedicated RV support devices include pulmonary artery balloon counterpulsation to reduce RV afterload, which required surgical implantation and, thus, had limited clinical application.[42] By the early 1990s, continuous-flow RVADs demonstrated better hemodynamic support and clinical outcomes compared with pulsatile devices for right ventricular failure (RVF).[43] Second- and third-generation surgical devices now include rotodynamic pumps that transferred rotational kinetic energy to the bloodstream and involved either multiple moving parts (impeller and bearings) or a single moving part (impeller), respectively.[41]

Percutaneously delivered assist devices that specifically address RV failure are relatively new. Historically, percutaneous mechanical support for RVF has been limited to the IABP. Nordhaug and colleagues[44] performed one of the few preclinical studies examining the impact of IABP use in a model of acute RV failure caused by microembolization of the RCA. In this study, IABP activation caused a small but statistically significant increase in systemic mean arterial pressure, total cardiac output, and biventricular stroke volume, while reducing both LV and RV afterload. Furthermore, a trend toward increased RCA flow was observed with IABP application. These data support the use of IABPs in the setting of acute RVMI; however, the hemodynamic impact is small and do not provide optimal RV unloading.[44]

In 2006, the first successful implantation of a percutaneously delivered RVAD in the setting of RV failure after AMI[45] using the TandemHeart centrifugal flow pump was reported (Fig. 3). Since then, the TandemHeart RVAD (TH-RVAD) has been implanted for RV failure in the setting of AMI,[46] post-LVAD implantation,[14] severe pulmonary hypertension,[47] and cardiac rejection after

Fig. 3. Deployment options for the TandemHeart RVAD. PA, pulmonary artery; RA, right atrium. (*Courtesy of* CardiacAssist, Pittsburgh, PA; with permission.)

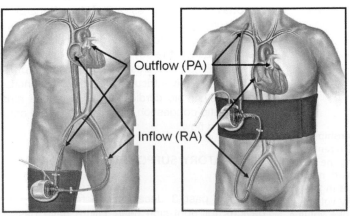

Femoral - Femoral   Internal Jugular – Femoral

orthotopic heart transplantation.[48] As a centrifugal pump that generates continuous flow with a minimal, low-amplitude pulsatile component, the TH-RVAD may more closely approximate native RV function and may have hemodynamic benefits over the more commonly used, surgically placed, pulsatile RVADs. Furthermore, the percutaneous application of a mechanical circulatory support device provides the opportunity for early intervention in the cascade of refractory RV failure without the need for surgery.

Other centrifugal pumps include the Centrimag (Thoratec Corporation, Pleasanton, CA), Rotaflow (Maquet, Rastatt, Germany), and Bio-Medicus (Medtronic, Inc, Minneapolis, MN) pumps (**Fig. 4**), which are more commonly implanted surgically or used to provide flow for venoarterial ECMO (VA-ECMO). VA-ECMO is used to enhance systemic oxygenation during cardiorespiratory collapse or to provide hemodynamic support in isolated RV or biventricular failure.[49–51] The major effect of VA-ECMO is to displace blood volume from the venous to the arterial circulation. As a result, a reduction in both RV and LV volumes can be observed with a concomitant increase in LV afterload. This increase in afterload is in contrast to left atrial-to-femoral artery bypass pumps because there is no direct venting of the LV with VA-ECMO. For this reason, some operators have combined VA-ECMO with the use of the Impella 2.5 to reduce any negative effects of increased LV afterload during VA-ECMO use.[52] Advantages of VA-ECMO include the relative ease of insertion and the ability to support systemic oxygenation.

More recently, the Impella RP axial-flow catheter has been developed and is currently undergoing evaluation as a support option for RV failure (**Fig. 5**).[53] A premarket clinical feasibility evaluation has been initiated at several sites in Canada and Europe in patients experiencing RVF in different clinical settings. Indications for use at the time of this submission included RVF after heart transplant,[2] RVF after cardiac surgery,[1] RVF after LVAD implantation,[2] and RVF after AMI.[1] All patients were in cardiogenic shock before the Impella RP implant. The percutaneous implant of the device was feasible and successful in 100% of the patients. The support time ranged from 1 to 9 days, with more than 60% of the patients being supported for longer than 4 days (median of 6.5 days) and explanted on RV recovery. The average flow was 3.9 L/min. Overall, the 30-day survival was 83%. Whether axial or centrifugal flow pumps provide better support for RV failure remains unknown. One potential advantage of centrifugal flow pumps is the ability to splice an oxygenator into the circuit and, thereby, provide ECMO support while unloading the RV, whereas an advantage of the Impella RP may be the ability to deploy the device using a single venous access site.

BIVENTRICULAR FAILURE

Biventricular failure is a primary determinant of poor outcomes in cardiogenic shock.[54] Persistent multiorgan failure often complicates biventricular failure and is a relative contraindication for surgical VAD placement. Recently, experience with

Pulastile Pumps

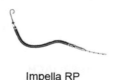

Intra-aortic Balloon Pump

Axial-Flow Pumps

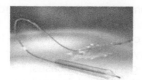

Impella RP

Centrifugal Pumps

Percutaneous/Surgical or VA-ECMO

TandemHeart

Surgical or VA-ECMO

RotaFlow   Centrimag   Biomedicus

Fig. 4. Percutaneous circulatory support devices for RV failure. VA-ECMO, venoarterial ECMO. (*Courtesy of* CardiacAssist, Pittsburgh, PA; with permission.)

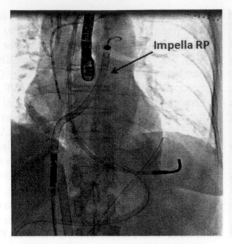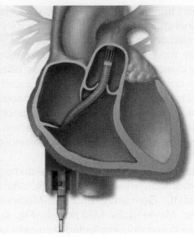

Fig. 5. The Impella RP axial-flow catheter. ([right] *Courtesy of* Abiomed Inc., Danvers, MA; with permission.)

percutaneously deployed circulatory support devices for biventricular failure has been growing[55]; however, the optimal strategy remains poorly understood. A recent study compared the effects of VA-ECMO, the TandemHeart left atrial-to-femoral artery bypass pump, and the Impella 2.5 LP device in a preclinical model of biventricular failure induced by acute ventricular fibrillation. In this study, mean arterial pressure was best supported with VA-ECMO, followed by the Tandem-Heart device, and with minimal support provided by the Impella 2.5 LP catheter unless norepinephrine was concomitantly administered.[56,57] In contrast, several studies have shown excellent hemodynamic support with the combined use of the Impella 5.0 or 2.5 LP devices for support of the left side of the heart with either a TH-RVAD or VA-ECMO for support of the right side of the heart.[57,58] As mechanical support options continue to develop, providing dedicated support of the right and left side of the heart may become more common in cases of refractory biventricular failure.

PREPROCEDURE PLANNING

Early identification of clinically significant RV failure is a critical aspect of preprocedural planning.[59] Clinical examination and laboratory findings include signs of poor systemic perfusion, elevated jugular venous pressures, and congestive hepatopathy. Echocardiographic evaluation of RV failure includes measurement of RV systolic function, dilatation grade, severity of tricuspid regurgitation, and quantitative assessment of the tricuspid annular plane systolic excursion value. Invasive measures of hemodynamic indices suggestive of RV failure include a central venous pressure greater

than 16 mm Hg, right atrial–to–pulmonary capillary wedge pressure ratio greater than 0.8 for AMI and 0.63 for post-LVAD failure, and an RV stroke work index less than 450 (units). More recently, the authors developed the pulmonary artery pulsatility index (PAPi) as a simple measure of RV failure without the need for an estimate of stroke volume. In several studies, a PAPi less than 1.0 correlated with severe RV failure.[25] Once identified, initial management includes urgent coronary revascularization, inotropic therapy, inhaled nitric oxide, and IABP support. In RV failure, therapy with a percutaneous RVAD should be considered soon after initial resuscitative efforts have failed. No definite algorithms for percutaneous mechanical RV support with a TH-RVAD have been developed.

PREPARATION AND PATIENT POSITIONING

Unlike conventional therapy for cardiogenic shock in acute RVMI with an IABP, the TH-RVAD provides centrifugal flow from the RA to the main pulmonary artery (PA), thereby bypassing a poorly functioning RV. In most cases, TH-RVAD cannulas are implanted via both femoral veins. Two cannulas are available in 62-cm and 72-cm lengths. Right internal jugular (IJ) cannulation of the main PA can be used when the distance from the femoral vein to the fifth intercostal space (ICS) exceeds 58 cm or if femoral venous access is limited by infection, thrombosis, or inferior vena caval filters (**Fig. 6**). Cannula lengths and vessel tortuosity may limit left IJ access. Standard patient positioning for cardiac catheterization is recommended.

PROCEDURAL APPROACH

For LV support, the TandemHeart centrifugal pump requires placement of 21-F inflow cannula

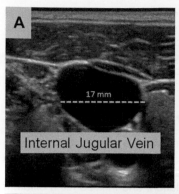

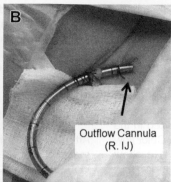

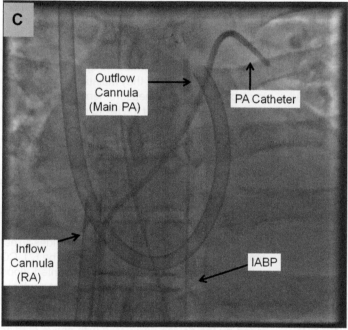

Fig. 6. TH-RVAD. (*A*) Ultrasound image of the right IJ vein before deployment of a TH-RVAD. (*B*) Appearance of the incision site and cannula placement in the right IJ vein. (*C*) Final fluoroscopic image of the TH-RVAD inflow and outflow cannulas in the main pulmonary artery (PA) and right atrium (RA). A PA catheter and IABP are also shown. (*Courtesy of* CardiacAssist, Pittsburgh, PA; with permission.)

(CardiacAssist Inc, Pittsburgh, PA) extending from the femoral vein, across the interatrial septum, into the left atrium. A second 15-F to 17-F outflow cannula is placed into a femoral artery. For RV support, a 21-F inflow cannula is instead positioned in the RA with a second 21-F outflow cannula inserted into the main PA. For TH-RVAD deployment, venous access is ideally achieved using vascular ultrasound to avoid inadvertent penetration of the femoral or carotid artery. For bifemoral cannulation, the right femoral vein is commonly used for the placement of the outflow cannula into the main PA and the left femoral vein is for inflow cannula deployment into the RA. For the right IJ approach, the outflow cannula is placed into the main PA via the IJ and the RA-inflow cannula is placed via a femoral vein (see **Fig. 3**).

To deploy the outflow cannula, a standard PA catheter is positioned into the main PA. Unfractionated

heparin should be administered with a goal-activated clotting time of 250 to 350 ms during cannula deployment. After recording baseline hemodynamic indices, the PA catheter is exchanged for a multipurpose catheter (MPC) using an exchange-length J-tipped wire. Once the MPC is positioned in a first- or second-order branch of the PA, an exchange length, reinforced 0.038 J-tipped wire (ie, Amplatz SuperStiff [Boston Scientific, Miami, FL]) is advanced into the PA and the MPC is removed. The venous puncture site is then serially dilated with 7-, 10-, and 12-F dilators, followed by final dilation with a graded 14- to 21-F dilator that is provided with the TH-RVAD kit (Video 1). Liberal blunt dissection with forceps may be required to optimize cannula deployment. Once the venous puncture is dilated, the 21-F cannula, with the obturator in place, is advanced into the main PA over the reinforced 0.038 inches wire (Video 2). When removing the wire and obturator, first pull the wire back into the obturator, then bring both wire and obturator out of the cannula as a single unit. A second operator must be prepared to clamp the 21-F cannula immediately after removal of the obturator using standard perfusion tubing clamps (Video 3). Optimal positioning of the outflow cannula is confirmed by fluoroscopy and transesophageal echocardiography in the catheterization laboratory. The outflow cannula tip should be visualized in the main PA above the pulmonic valve plane. Color flow Doppler echocardiography can be used to show flow above the pulmonic valve (**Fig. 7**). For inflow cannula deployment, a standard 0.038 inches J-tipped wire is placed into the right atrium. After dilating the venous access site, the 21-F inflow cannula and obturator are deployed in similar fashion to the outflow cannula followed by clamping.

Priming of the centrifugal pump can be performed anytime during the procedure. In most instances, the pump is primed immediately after successful deployment of the outflow cannula into the main PA. Protocols for pump priming are described in the operating manual for the TH-RVAD. Once the pump is primed, wet-to-wet connections are made between the appropriate cannulas and tubing segments of the pump with meticulous attention to de-airing. Three of the 4 clamps are released and the pump activated, followed by immediate release of the final clamp (see Video 3).

IMMEDIATE POSTPROCEDURAL CARE

Often a PA catheter is deployed after device activation to monitor patients' hemodynamic response. Careful positioning of the distal PA catheter tip in the proximal segment of the right or left PA is required. The PA catheter balloon is left deflated to avoid antegrade migration of the catheter. Once the TH-RVAD is activated, both inflow and outflow cannulas are stabilized using sutures and adhesive pads. The centrifugal pump is stabilized using a Velcro holster. All cannula depths

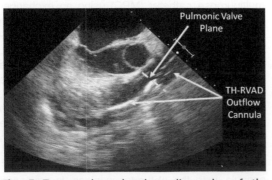

Fig. 7. Transesophageal echocardiography of the TH-RVAD outflow cannula across the RV outflow tract and pulmonic valve plane.

should be recorded and marked in centimeters at the skin insertion site for future reference. Patients are then transported out of the catheterization laboratory with careful attention to all cannula depths to avoid displacement out of the main PA or right atrium.

REHABILITATION AND RECOVERY

After TH-RVAD insertion and activation, ongoing management of RV failure includes continued inotropic and vasopressor support as needed, mechanical ventilation, and inhaled nitric oxide. If an IABP was deployed before TH-RVAD insertion, the IABP may be left activated in place and is not likely to interfere with the function of the TH-RVAD. Monitoring hemodynamic conditions after device placement is critical to guide therapy. In the authors' institution, they maintain a PA catheter in place for ongoing measurements of filling pressures of the right side of the heart, pulmonary artery pulsatility, and Fick-derived cardiac output measurements. The authors further monitor the degree of hemodynamic support provided by the TH-RVAD by measuring total cardiac output (T-CO) after device implantation using the Fick method and comparing this value with flow (F) through the device as measured by a probe attached to the outflow cannula (provided in the TH-RVAD kit). The difference between T-CO and F provides an estimate of native cardiac output (nCO). The F/T-CO ratio represented the degree of augmented blood flow generated by the percutaneous right ventricular support device (pRVSD). Using these values, the authors can track the magnitude of support provided by the device compared with native cardiac function over time (**Fig. 8**). Once nCO approximates T-CO with minimal support from the TH-RVAD, the authors consider device withdrawal. Inotropic and vasopressor support may be required during weaning and after device removal.

As is the case with most support devices, hemodynamic stability and adequate systemic perfusion at a low device setting often indicates that device removal is feasible. At the time of device removal, both inflow and outflow cannulas are clamped and the device is turned off. Within minutes of device deactivation, the outflow and inflow cannulas are removed with manual compression over both venous access sites to achieve hemostasis. In anticoagulated patients, prolonged compression may be required to achieve optimal hemostasis.

CLINICAL STUDIES

At present, minimal data exploring the clinical utility of percutaneous RV support devices exist.

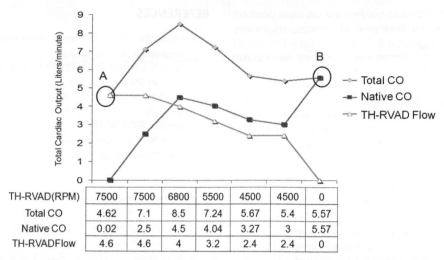

TH-RVAD(RPM)	7500	7500	6800	5500	4500	4500	0
Total CO	4.62	7.1	8.5	7.24	5.67	5.4	5.57
Native CO	0.02	2.5	4.5	4.04	3.27	3	5.57
TH-RVADFlow	4.6	4.6	4	3.2	2.4	2.4	0

Fig. 8. *The Journal of Heart and Lung Transplantation* figure for calculation of percent augmentation. Changes in T-CO relative to augmented flow generated by the TH-RVAD over time during device weaning in a single representative patient. Each time point represents 1 day beginning with initiation of TH-RVAD at 7500 rotations per minute (RPMs). As T-CO improves during maximal TH-RVAD support, RPMs are reduced and native CO improves over time. At TH-RVAD initiation (A), T-CO is completely supported by the TH-RVAD. At device deactivation (B), T-CO matches native CO. (*Data from* Kapur N, Paruchuri V, Korabathina R, et al. Effects of a percutaneous mechanical circulatory support device for medically refractory right ventricular failure. J Heart Lung Transplant 2011;30(12):1365.)

Several studies have shown the potential benefits of centrifugal flow pumps in RV failure using surgical and hybridized surgical-percutaneous deployment with the Centrimag[60] and the Rotaflow[61] pumps, respectively. The authors recently reported their single-center experience with fully percutaneous deployment of the TH-RVSD in 9 patients with medically refractory RV failure and identified that compared with preprocedural values, mean arterial pressure (57 ± 7 vs 75 ± 19, $P<.05$), right atrial pressure (22 ± 3 vs 15 ± 6, $P<.05$), cardiac index (1.5 ± 0.4 vs 2.3 ± 0.5, $P<.05$), mixed venous oxygen saturation (40 ± 14 vs 58 ± 4, $P<.05$), and RV stroke work (3.4 ± 3.9 vs 9.7 ± 6.8, $P<.05$) improved significantly within 24 hours of TH-RVSD implantation. In-hospital mortality among 9 patients was 44% (n = 4). The time from admission to TH-RVSD placement was lower in patients who survived to hospital discharge (0.9 ± 0.8 vs 4.8 ± 3.5 days, $P = .04$, survivors vs nonsurvivors). In this report, no mechanical complications were observed during or after device implantation, suggesting that TH-RVSD is clinically feasible and may not be associated with excess risk.[59]

More recently, the TandemHeart in RIght VEntricular support (THRIVE) study was a retrospective, observational registry of 46 patients receiving a TH-RVAD for RV failure in 8 tertiary care centers in the United States. The central finding of this report was that implantation of the

TH-RVAD is clinically feasible via both surgical and percutaneous routes and is associated with acute hemodynamic improvement in RV failure across a broad variety of clinical presentations. This study also identified that evaluation of RV failure in real-world practice did not always involve quantitative measures of RV function and, further, does not always include comprehensive evaluation and management of concomitant LV dysfunction. In-hospital mortality varied widely among different indications for mechanical RV support and was lowest among patients with RV failure in the setting of AMI or after LVAD implantation. Increased age, biventricular failure, and Thrombolysis In Myocardial Infarction (TIMI) major bleeding were more commonly observed in patients not surviving to hospital discharge.[62]

Clinical experience with the Impella RP axial flow catheter remains limited at this time.

POTENTIAL COMPLICATIONS

Because the TH-RVSD provides centrifugal flow from the right atrium to the main pulmonary artery (PA), penetration of cannulas into the heart is required to bypass a poorly functioning RV. Close monitoring for evidence of cannula migration is essential and can be prevented by marking cannula depths at the skin incision site, minimizing patient mobility and stabilizing cannulas during patient transport. Echocardiographic and daily chest radiographs to confirm the cannula position also reduce the likelihood of cannula migration. Antegrade migration into a secondary branch of the pulmonary arteries could present as hypoxic respiratory failure, hemothorax, hemoptysis, decreased cardiac output, and an acute decrease in TH-RVAD flows. Retrograde migration into the RV may result in decreased cardiac output because of tricuspid regurgitation, reduced TH-RVAD flows, or ventricular arrhythmia. Although antegrade or retrograde cannula migration are possible, no institutions in the THRIVE study reported migration as a device-associated complication. TIMI major bleeding was the most common complication associated with the TH-RVSD and is likely secondary to the need for continuous anticoagulation and sheathless deployment of the device cannulas. Bleeding is best controlled by close monitoring of anticoagulation and minimizing patient movement while on support. Mechanical complications associated with the TH-RVSD were rare and included isolated cases of injury to the main PA during surgical deployment only and an isolated case of retroperitoneal bleed associated with peripheral venous cannulation. The development of deep venous thrombosis was reported in 3 cases despite required anticoagulation during device support and may be caused by severe multiorgan dysfunction or partial obstruction of venous flow by cannulas in the inferior vena cava.[62]

SUMMARY

RV failure is a major cause of global morbidity and mortality. As the population of patients with heart failure continues to grow, the need for percutaneously delivered RV-dedicated circulatory support devices is becoming more apparent. Percutaneous RV support devices now represent an important approach to the management of RV failure and provide an opportunity to rapidly deliver mechanical support as either a bridge to definitive therapy or recovery as advances in coronary intervention, cardiac surgery, pulmonary hypertension, transplant medicine, and VAD technology provide more options for patients surviving cardiogenic shock. As experience with RV devices grows, their role in the armamentarium of the mechanical therapies for RV failure will depend less on the technical ability to place the device and more on improved algorithms for patient selection, patient and device monitoring, and weaning protocols.

SUPPLEMENTARY DATA

Supplementary data related to this article can be found online at http://dx.doi.org/10.1016/j.iccl.2013.04.001.

REFERENCES

1. Lopez-Sendon J. The heart failure epidemic. Medicographia 2011;33:363–9.
2. Ghio S, Gavazzi A, Campana C, et al. Independent and additive prognostic value of right ventricular systolic function and pulmonary artery pressure in patients with chronic heart failure. J Am Coll Cardiol 2001;37:183–8.
3. Zehender M, Kasper W, Kauder E, et al. Right ventricular infarction as an independent predictor of prognosis after acute inferior myocardial infarction. N Engl J Med 1993;328:981–8.
4. Jacobs AK, Leopold JA, Bates E, et al. Cardiogenic shock caused by right ventricular infarction: a report from the SHOCK registry. J Am Coll Cardiol 2003;41:1273–9.
5. Budweiser S, Jörres RA, Riedl T, et al. Predictors of survival in COPD patients with chronic hypercapnic respiratory failure receiving noninvasive home ventilation. Chest 2007;131(6):1650–8.
6. Benza RL, Miller DP, Gomberg-Maitland M, et al. Predicting survival in pulmonary arterial hypertension: insights from the Registry to Evaluate Early and Long-Term Pulmonary Arterial Hypertension Disease Management (REVEAL). Circulation 2010;122:164–72.
7. Haddad F, Peterson T, Fuh E, et al. Characteristics and outcome after hospitalization for acute right heart failure in patients with pulmonary arterial hypertension. Circ Heart Fail 2011;4:692–9.
8. Apostolakis S, Konstantinides S. The right ventricle in health and disease: insights into physiology, pathophysiology and diagnostic management. Cardiology 2012;121(4):263–73.
9. Sanchez O, Planquette B, Roux A, et al. Triaging in pulmonary embolism. Semin Respir Crit Care Med 2012;33:156–62.
10. McLaughlin VV, Archer SL, Badesch DB, et al. ACCF/AHA 2009 expert consensus document on pulmonary hypertension a report of the American College of Cardiology Foundation Task Force on Expert Consensus Documents and the American Heart Association developed in collaboration with the American College of Chest Physicians; American Thoracic Society, Inc; and the Pulmonary Hypertension Association. J Am Coll Cardiol 2009; 53:1573–619.
11. Bursi F, McNallan SM, Redfield MM, et al. Pulmonary pressures and death in heart failure a community study. J Am Coll Cardiol 2012;59(3): 222–31.
12. Dandel M, Lehmkuhl HB, Knosalla C, et al. Impact of different long-term maintenance immunosuppressive therapy strategies on patients' outcome after heart transplantation. Transpl Immunol 2010; 23(3):93–103.

13. Vlahakes GJ. Right ventricular failure after cardiac surgery. Cardiol Clin 2012;30(2):283–9.

14. Takagaki M, Wurzer C, Wade R, et al. Successful conversion of TandemHeart left ventricular assist device to right ventricular assist device after implantation of a HeartMate XVE. Ann Thorac Surg 2008;86:1677–9.

15. Masci PG, Francone M, Desmet W, et al. Right ventricular ischemic injury in patients with acute ST-segment elevation myocardial infarction: characterization with cardiovascular magnetic resonance. Circulation 2010;122(14):1405–12.

16. Engström AE, Vis MM, Bouma BJ, et al. Right ventricular dysfunction is an independent predictor for mortality in ST-elevation myocardial infarction patients presenting with cardiogenic shock on admission. Eur J Heart Fail 2010;12(3):276–82.

17. Alam M, Wardell J, Andersson E, et al. Right ventricular function in patients with first inferior myocardial infarction: assessment by tricuspid annular motion and tricuspid annular velocity. Am Heart J 2000;139(4):710–5.

18. O'Rourke RA, Dell'Italia LJ. Diagnosis and management of right ventricular myocardial infarction. Curr Probl Cardiol 2004;29:6–47.

19. Metha S, Eikelboom J, Natarajan M. Impact of right ventricular involvement on mortality and morbidity in patients with inferior myocardial infarction. J Am Coll Cardiol 2001;37:37–43.

20. Piazza G, Goldhaber SZ. The acutely decompensated right ventricle: pathways for diagnosis and management. Chest 2005;128:1836–52.

21. Haddad F, Doyle R, Murphy DJ, et al. Right ventricular function in cardiovascular disease, part II: pathophysiology, clinical importance, and management of right ventricular failure. Circulation 2008;117:1717–31.

22. Kelly RG. Building the right ventricle. Circ Res 2007;100(7):943–5.

23. Chin KM, Coghlan G. Characterizing the right ventricle: advancing our knowledge. Am J Cardiol 2012;110(Suppl 6):3S–8S. http://dx.doi.org/10.1016/j.amjcard.2012.06.010.

24. Greyson CR. The right ventricle and pulmonary circulation: basic concepts. Rev Esp Cardiol 2010;63:81–95.

25. Korabathina R, Heffernan KS, Paruchuri V, et al. The pulmonary artery pulsatility index identifies severe right ventricular dysfunction in acute inferior myocardial infarction. Catheter Cardiovasc Interv 2011. http://dx.doi.org/10.1002/ccd.23309.

26. Redington AN, Rigby ML, Shinebourne EA, et al. Changes in the pressure-volume relation of the right ventricle when its loading conditions are modified. Br Heart J 1990;63(1):45–9.

27. Brown KA, Ditchey RV. Human right ventricular end-systolic pressure-volume relation defined by maximal elastance. Circulation 1988;78(1):81–91.

28. Asanoi H, Sasayama S, Kameyama T. Ventriculoarterial coupling in normal and failing heart in humans. Circ Res 1989;65(2):483–93 [Erratum in: Circ Res 1990;66:1170].

29. Kapur N, Aronovitz M, Blanton R, et al. The ventriculo-ventricular coupling index: a novel approach to assessing biventricular function. Circ Res 2012;111:A89.

30. Dell'Italia LJ, Starling MR, Crawford MH, et al. Right ventricular infarction: identification by hemodynamic measurements before and after volume loading and correlation with noninvasive techniques. J Am Coll Cardiol 1984;4:931–9.

31. Smiseth OA, Kingma I, Refsum H, et al. The pericardial hypothesis: a mechanism of acute shifts of the left ventricular diastolic pressure-volume relation. Clin Physiol 1985;5(5):403–15.

32. Tyberg JV, Smith ER. Ventricular diastole and the role of the pericardium. Herz 1990;15(6):354–61.

33. Tyberg JV, Belenkie I, Manyari DE, et al. Ventricular interaction and venous capacitance modulate left ventricular preload. Can J Cardiol 1996;12(10):1058–64.

34. Champion HC, Michelakis ED, Hassoun PM. Comprehensive invasive and noninvasive approach to the right ventricle-pulmonary circulation unit: state of the art and clinical and research implications. Circulation 2009;120(11):992–1007.

35. Badesch DB, Champion HC, Sanchez MA, et al. Diagnosis and assessment of pulmonary arterial hypertension. J Am Coll Cardiol 2009;54(Suppl 1):S55–66.

36. Hemnes AR, Champion HC. Right heart function and haemodynamics in pulmonary hypertension. Int J Clin Pract Suppl 2008;(160):11–9.

37. Borlaug BA, Kass DA. Invasive hemodynamic assessment in heart failure. Heart Fail Clin 2009;5(2):217–28.

38. Greyson CR. Pathophysiology of right ventricular failure. Crit Care Med 2008;36:S57–65.

39. Goldstein JA. Acute right ventricular infarction: insights for the interventional era. Curr Probl Cardiol 2012;37(12):533–57.

40. John R, Lee S, Eckman P, et al. Right ventricular failure–a continuing problem in patients with left ventricular assist device support. J Cardiovasc Transl Res 2010;3(6):604–11.

41. Patel SM, Allaire PE, Wood HG, et al. Methods of failure and reliability assessment for mechanical heart pumps. Artif Organs 2005;29(1):15–25.

42. Flege JB Jr, Wright CB, Reisinger TJ. Successful balloon counterpulsation for right ventricular failure. Ann Thorac Surg 1984;37(2):167–8.

43. Taylor AJ, Edwards FH, Macon MG. A comparative evaluation of pulmonary artery balloon counterpulsation and a centrifugal flow pump in an

experimental model of right ventricular infarction. J Extra Corpor Technol 1990;22(2):85–90.

44. Nordhaug D, Steensrud T, Muller S, et al. Intraaortic balloon pumping improves hemodynamics and right ventricular efficiency in acute ischemic right ventricular failure. Ann Thorac Surg 2004;78(4): 1426–32.

45. Atiemo AD, Conte JV, Heldman AW. Resuscitation and recovery from acute right ventricular failure using a percutaneous right ventricular assist device. Catheter Cardiovasc Interv 2006;68(1):78–82.

46. Prutkin JM, Strote JA, Stout KK. Percutaneous right ventricular assist device as support for cardiogenic shock due to right ventricular infarction. J Invasive Cardiol 2008;20(7):E215–6.

47. Rajdev S, Benza R, Misra V. Use of Tandem Heart as a temporary hemodynamic support option for severe pulmonary artery hypertension complicated by cardiogenic shock. J Invasive Cardiol 2007; 19(8):E226–9.

48. Bajona P, Salizzoni S, Brann SH, et al. Prolonged use of right ventricular assist device for refractory graft failure following orthotopic heart transplantation. J Thorac Cardiovasc Surg 2010;139(3):e53–4.

49. Scherer M, Sirat AS, Moritz A, et al. Extracorporeal membrane oxygenation as perioperative right ventricular support in patients with biventricular failure undergoing left ventricular assist device implantation. Eur J Cardiothorac Surg 2011;39(6):939–44 [discussion: 944].

50. Ouweneel DM, Henriques JP. Percutaneous cardiac support devices for cardiogenic shock: current indications and recommendations. Heart 2012;98(16): 1246–54.

51. Kar B, Basra SS, Shah NR, et al. Percutaneous circulatory support in cardiogenic shock: interventional bridge to recovery. Circulation 2012;125(14):1809–17.

52. Kawashima D, Gojo S, Nishimura T, et al. Left ventricular mechanical support with Impella provides more ventricular unloading in heart failure than extracorporeal membrane oxygenation. ASAIO J 2011;57(3):169–76.

53. Cheung A, Freed D, Hunziker P, et al. TCT-371 first clinical evaluation of a novel percutaneous right ventricular assist device: the Impella RP. J Am Coll Cardiol 2012;60(17S):B106.

54. Potapov EV, Stepanenko A, Kukucka M, et al. Prediction of survival in patients with cardiogenic shock and multiorgan failure treated with biventricular assist device. ASAIO J 2010;56(4): 273–8.

55. Kar B, Gregoric ID, Basra SS, et al. The percutaneous ventricular assist device in severe refractory cardiogenic shock. J Am Coll Cardiol 2011;57(6): 688–96.

56. Ostadal P, Mlcek M, Holy F, et al. Direct comparison of percutaneous circulatory support systems in specific hemodynamic conditions in a porcine model. Circ Arrhythm Electrophysiol 2012;5(6): 1202–6.

57. Rajagopal V, Steahr G, Wilmer CI, et al. A novel percutaneous mechanical biventricular bridge to recovery in severe cardiac allograft rejection. J Heart Lung Transplant 2010;29(1):93–5.

58. Chaparro SV, Badheka A, Marzouka GR, et al. Combined use of Impella left ventricular assist device and extracorporeal membrane oxygenation as a bridge to recovery in fulminant myocarditis. ASAIO J 2012;58(3):285–7.

59. Kapur N, Paruchuri V, Korabathina R, et al. Effects of a percutaneous mechanical circulatory support device for medically refractory right ventricular failure. J Heart Lung Transplant 2011;30(12):1360–7. http://dx.doi.org/10.1016/j.healun.2011.07.005.

60. Hsu PL, Parker J, Egger C, et al. Mechanical circulatory support for right heart failure: current technology and future outlook. Artif Organs 2012;36(4): 332–47. http://dx.doi.org/10.1111/j.1525-1594.2011.01366.x.

61. Loor G, Khani-Hanjani A, Gonzalez-Stawinski GV. Use of RotaFlow (MAQUET) for temporary right ventricular support during implantation of HeartMate II left ventricular assist device. ASAIO J 2012;58(3):275–7. http://dx.doi.org/10.1097/MAT.0b013e318247088c.

62. Kapur N, Paruchuri V, Jagannathan A, et al. Mechanical circulatory support for right ventricular failure. JCHF 2013;1(2):127–34.

Percutaneous Assist Devices for Left Ventricular Shock

Sukhdeep S. Basra, MD, MPH[a],*, Pranav Loyalka, MD[b],
Igor Gregoric, MD[b], Ravi S. Hira, MD[a], Biswajit Kar, MD[b]

KEYWORDS

- Shock • Heart-assist device • Balloon • Hemodynamics • Heart failure • Resuscitation

KEY POINTS

- Percutaneous ventricular assist devices offer a rapid, minimally invasive, adequate, and effective means of support in patients with left ventricular shock not responsive to conventional therapies.
- Their use should be tailored to the patient's hemodynamic status, end-organ function, amount of cardiac support needed, as well as comorbidities.
- There is a lack of consensus on current applications, device selection, and cost-effective use of these devices.
- Further randomized trials are needed to evaluate these devices and establish the ideal device for different patient subgroups.

INTRODUCTION

Over the last 2 decades, percutaneous ventricular assist devices (PVADs) have rapidly grown to be safe and effective tools for the management of left ventricular cardiogenic shock (LVCS). In patients who fail to respond to standard medical therapies (including vasopressors and/or inotropes), PVADs can effectively unload the ventricles and reverse end-organ dysfunction. Although there is a lack of randomized trials, the use of PVADs is currently recommended by the American College of Cardiology Foundation, American Heart Association, and Society for Cardiovascular Angiography and Interventions for hemodynamically unstable patients with cardiogenic shock (CS) after ST-segment elevation myocardial infarctions (STEMI), who fail to stabilize with pharmacologic therapy (class I, level of evidence: B) based on superior hemodynamic improvements seen in patients implanted with these devices. It is also recommended for elective use for hemodynamic support during high-risk percutaneous coronary intervention (PCI; Class IIb, level of evidence: C) (**Table 1**).[1] Here, the currently available PVADs for LVCS, literature supporting their use, indications, complications, and future directions are reviewed.

CARDIOGENIC SHOCK

CS is a result of end-organ hypoperfusion due to left-ventricular, right-ventricular, or biventricular myocardial dysfunction resulting in systolic and/or diastolic myocardial pump failure.[2] The most common cause of CS continues to be myocardial infarction (MI) of the left ventricle (LV), resulting in left ventricular shock. CS complicates 8.6% of STEMI[3] and 2.5% of non–STEMI.[4] Common causes of LVCS are listed in **Box 1**.

Funding Resources: None.
Disclosures: None.
[a] Department of Cardiology, Baylor College of Medicine, One Baylor Plaza, Houston, TX 77030, USA;
[b] Department of Cardiology, Center for Advanced Heart Failure, University of Texas Health Science Center at Houston, 6410 Fannin Street, Suite # 370, Houston, TX 77030, USA
* Corresponding author.
E-mail address: basra@bcm.edu

Intervent Cardiol Clin 2 (2013) 457–468
http://dx.doi.org/10.1016/j.iccl.2013.03.005
2211-7458/13/$ – see front matter © 2013 Elsevier Inc. All rights reserved.

Table 1
American College of Cardiology Foundation, American Heart Association, and Society for Cardiovascular Angiography and Interventions (ACC/AHA/SCAI) and ESC/EACT guidelines on IABP and PVAD for cardiogenic shock and high-risk PCI

Indication	Assist Device	ESC/EACT Guidelines	ACCF/AHA/SCAI Guidelines
Cardiogenic shock	IABP	IABP insertion is recommended in patients with hemodynamic instability (particularly those in cardiogenic shock and with mechanical complications)	A hemodynamic support device is recommended for patients with cardiogenic shock after STEMI who do not quickly stabilize with pharmacologic therapy
		Class IIb (level of evidence)	Class IIa (level of evidence B)
	TandemHeart	Routine use of percutaneous centrifugal pumps is not recommended	
		Class IIb (level of evidence C)	Class IIb (level of evidence C)
	Impella	No recommendation	No recommendation
	ECMO	ECMO implantation should be considered for temporary support in patients with AHF with potential for functional recovery following revascularization	
		No recommendation	
High-risk PCI	IABP	The systematic use of balloon counterpulsation, in the absence of hemodynamic impairment, is not recommended	Elective insertion of an appropriate hemodynamic support device as an adjunct to PCI may be reasonable in carefully selected high-risk patients
		Class III (level of evidence B)	Class IIb (level of evidence C)
	TandemHeart	Routine use of percutaneous centrifugal pumps is not recommended	
		Class III (level of evidence B)	
	Impella	No recommendation	No recommendation
	ECMO	No recommendation	No recommendation

From Ouweneel DM, Henriques JP. Percutaneous cardiac support devices for cardiogenic shock: current indications and recommendations. Heart 2012;98(16):1246–54; with permission.

Box 1
Common causes of LVS

MI without mechanical complications

MI with mechanical complications (ventricular septal rupture, or papillary muscle/chordal rupture)

Acute decompensation of chronic heart failure

Acute myocarditis

Postcardiotomy

Takotsubo/stress-induced cardiomyopathy

Peripartum cardiomyopathy

Refractory arrhythmias

Cardiac tamponade

Acute rejection after orthotopic heart transplant

Hypertrophic cardiomyopathy with severe outflow obstruction

Aortic dissection complicated by acute severe aortic insufficiency and/or MI

At the bedside, CS is defined by both hemodynamic and clinical parameters. Clinical parameters include persistent hypotension (systolic blood pressure of <90 mm Hg for at least 30 minutes or the need for supportive measures to maintain a systolic blood pressure of ≥90 mm Hg) and end-organ hypoperfusion (cool extremities or a urine output of <30 mL per hour), whereas hemodynamic parameters include a cardiac index $<2.2 \, L \cdot min^{-1} \cdot m^{-2}$ and elevated filling pressures (pulmonary capillary wedge pressure >15 mm Hg).[5] Decreased perfusion and end-organ dysfunction lead to lactic acidosis, catecholamine, and neurohormonal release along with activation of systemic inflammatory and coagulation cascades, which eventually results in a downward spiral with further myocardial depression and hypoperfusion.

CS presents with a wide clinical spectrum ranging from preshock (significant risk of developing CS), mild CS (responsive to low-dose inotropes/vasopressors), profound CS (responsive to high-dose inotropes/vasopressors and intra-aortic balloon pump [IABP]), and severe refractory CS (SRCS; unresponsive to high-dose inotropes/vasopressors and IABP). Based on these definitions, an escalation of treatment protocols is recommended (**Fig. 1**).[2] The aim is to restore adequate perfusion and prevent end-organ dysfunction, thus breaking the downward spiral of untreated CS.

IABP Counterpulsation

IABP counterpulsation continues to be the most widely used mechanical assist device for CS because of LV failure. During diastole, balloon inflation occurs, which improves coronary and peripheral perfusion. Balloon inflation is followed by balloon deflation during systole, creating a suction effect and decreasing afterload, which augments left ventricular output. With IABP, cardiac output is augmented by up to 0.5 L/min.[6]

Data from the SHOCK trial registry suggested improved mortality in patients with MI who received IABP in addition to thrombolytic therapy or early revascularization with percutaneous transluminal coronary angioplasty/coronary artery bypass graft.[7] Similarly, the GUSTO-1 trial showed early institution of IABP and thrombolytic therapy in patients with acute myocardial infarction (AMI) complicated by CS was associated with a trend toward lower 30-day and 1-year all-cause mortality despite an increased risk of adverse events.[8] Analysis from the National Registry of Myocardial Infarction also demonstrated that IABP use in patients with AMI complicated by CS was associated with a significant mortality reduction when used in conjunction with thrombolytic therapy, but not with primary angioplasty.[9]

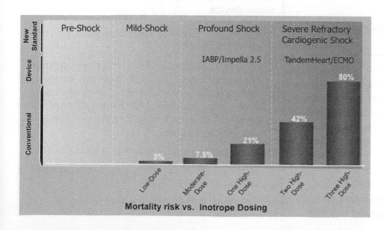

Fig. 1. Clinical spectrum of cardiogenic shock. ECMO, extracorporeal membrane oxygenation; IABP, intra-aortic balloon pressure. (*Adapted from* Samuels LE, Kaufman MS, Thomas MP, et al. Pharmacological criteria for ventricular assist device insertion following postcardiotomy shock: experience with the Abiomed BVS system. J Card Surg 1999;14:288–93; with permission.)

However, in a randomized controlled trial of patients with AMI and CS undergoing PCI, the addition of IABPs compared with medical therapy did not result in a significant improvement in multiorgan dysfunction syndrome, cardiac index, or systemic inflammatory activation.[10] A recent meta-analysis also suggested that despite a beneficial effect on hemodynamic parameters, IABPs do not have a mortality benefit.[11] Finally, Sjauw and colleagues[12] conducted a meta-analysis demonstrating no improvement in 30-day survival or LV ejection fraction, but an increased risk of stroke and bleeding complications with the use of IABP in patients with STEMI complicated by CS.

IABPs also continue to be the most commonly used PVAD support during high-risk PCI. However, the BCIS study demonstrated that elective initiation of IABP in patients undergoing high-risk PCI did not reduce the incidence of major adverse cardiac events (MACE).[13] The Counterpulsation to Reduce Infarct Size Pre-PCI Acute Myocardial Infarction randomized trial also failed to show any reduction in infarct size associated with the use of IABP therapy in 337 patients with anterior STEMI without shock.[14] The recently published IABP-SHOCK II trial in which 600 patients with LVCS complicating AMI were randomly assigned to either receive or not receive IABP in addition to early revascularization showed no significant difference in mortality, time to hemodynamic stabilization, or length of intensive care unit stay at 30 days.[15]

These studies have questioned the current role of IABP in patients with LVCS. There are considerable logistical and design challenges in conducting appropriate randomized trials to evaluate the efficacy of IABP in patients with LVCS and the results of the above studies must be interpreted with caution. IABP support alone may not be sufficient to change the outcomes in these patients and further therapies instituted while on IABP support may affect outcomes.

Surgically Implanted Temporary Ventricular Assist Devices

The next generations of ventricular assist devices (VADs) were temporary devices, which were surgically implanted and designed to provide full circulatory support. These temporary VADs included the Abiomed BVS System 5000 (Abiomed, Inc, Danvers, MA, USA), an external, automated, gravity-filled, pneumatically driven device with blood inflow from the left atrium returned to the thoracic aorta via transthoracic cannula insertion.

The Abiomed BVS System 5000 was followed by the next generation of surgically implanted external VADs, such as the CentriMag VAD (Levitronix, Waltham, MA, USA). These surgically implanted external VADs are magnetically levitated, continuous-flow, rotary pumps designed to minimize blood trauma and mechanical failure and were first used for postcardiotomy CS and as a bridge-to-decision in 2006.[16] A recent multicenter trial[17] showed it to have a low incidence of device-related complications and be an effective bridge-to-recovery device in patients with severe graft rejection after heart transplantation (1-year survival of 32%).[18] The cannulae can be inserted percutaneously.[19]

More recently, the Impella Recover 5.0 VAD (Abiomed Inc) was introduced. It is a catheter-mounted microaxial rotary pump inserted into the LV in a retrograde fashion via the femoral artery or axillary artery access after surgical cut-down and is capable of augmenting CO by 5.0 L/min. It has been effective as a bridge-to-transplant,[20] a bridge-to-bridge,[21] and as a bridge-to-recovery.[22,23]

Despite considerable improvement in morbidity and mortality associated with the use of surgically implanted short-term VADs, these devices are limited by the need for general anesthesia and delayed time to implantation in the operating room. PVADs were thus developed to overcome these limitations while maintaining full circulatory support.

PERCUTANEOUS LEFT VENTRICULAR ASSIST DEVICES

Box 2 demonstrates the most desirable features in a percutaneous LVAD. The current generation of PVADs includes the TandemHeart PVAD, the Impella Recover 2.5 PVAD, Impellac VAD, and percutaneous extracorporeal membrane oxygenation (ECMO) (**Table 2**):

Box 2
Ideal features of a percutaneous left ventricular assist device

1. Rapid and easy implantation via a percutaneous approach;

2. Effective and reliable circulatory support (flow) to adequately unload the impaired ventricles, maintain systemic perfusion pressure, and reverse end-organ dysfunction (even in the setting of increased systemic vascular resistance);

3. Easy/uncomplicated operation postinsertion;

4. Low complication rates (eg, limb ischemia, stroke, and hemolysis);

5. Easy weaning and removal

Table 2
Comparison of currently available PVADs

	IABP	TandemHeart	Impella 2.5	ImpellacVAD	ECMO
Pump mechanism	Pneumatic	Centrifugal	Axial	Axial	Centrifugal
Insertion	Retrograde 7–9-F balloon catheter into descending aorta via femoral artery	21-F inflow cannula into left atrium via femoral vein and transseptal puncture and 15/17-F outflow cannula into femoral artery	12-F catheter (13-F sheath) retrograde across aortic valve via femoral artery	14-F catheter placed retrogradely across the aortic valve via the femoral artery	18–31-F inflow cannula into right atrium via femoral vein and 15–22-F outflow cannula into descending aorta via femoral artery
Difficulty of insertion	+	++++	+++	+++	++
Degree of circulatory support (with ideal SVR)	+ (⇑ CO by 0.5 L/min)	+++ (⇑ CO by 3.5–4.5 L/min)	++ (⇑ CO by 2.5 L/min)	+++ (⇑ CO by 3.7 L/min)	++++ (⇑ CO to ≥4.5 L/min)
Implantation time	10 min	25–65 min	11–25 min	11–25 min	10–15 min
Limb ischemia risk	+	+++	++	++	++
Hemolysis	0	++	++++	+++	+++
Bleeding risk	+	+++	++	++	++++
510 K approval duration	Unspecified	6 h	6 h	6 h	6 h
Evidence of efficacy	Increased CO, coronary and peripheral perfusion. Decreased afterload	Increased CO, MAP, MVO2, and urine output. Decreased lactic acid, creatinine, and PCWP	Increased CO and MAP. Decreased lactic acid and PCWP	Increased CO and MAP. Decreased lactic acid and PCWP	Increased CO, MAP, and oxygenation

TandemHeart PVAD

The TandemHeart PVAD (CardiacAssist, Inc, Pittsburgh, PA, USA) is a left atrial-femoral bypass centrifugal pump capable of providing rapid short-term circulatory support up to 3.5 to 4.5 L/min of CO (**Fig. 2**). It is currently US Food and Drug Administration (FDA) approved for up to 6 hours of circulatory support.

In animal models of AMI and LVCS, Tandem-Heart PVAD restored endocardial and epicardial blood flow and was associated with substantial reduction in infarct size.[24] Burkhoff and colleagues compared IABP to TandemHeart PVAD in patients

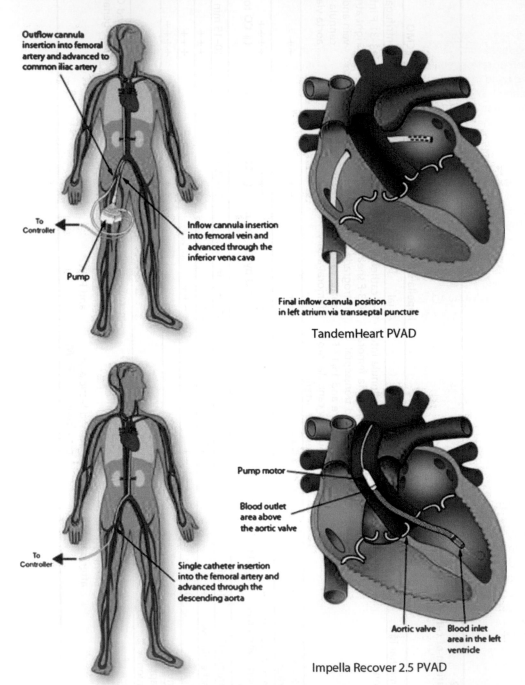

Fig. 2. Inflow/outflow cannulae configurations for the TandemHeart and Impella Recover 2.5 PVADs. (*From* Kar B, Basra SS, Shah NR, et al. Percutaneous circulatory support in cardiogenic shock: interventional bridge to recovery. Circulation 2012;125(14):1809–17; with permission.)

with CS and showed that it provided significantly better hemodynamic support than IABPs, with no significant difference in 30-day mortality and similar adverse events.[25] A subsequent randomized trial in patients with LVCS after AMI undergoing PCI demonstrated similar results with significant improvement in hemodynamic parameters and no difference in 30-day mortality. However, complications including severe bleeding and limb ischemia were encountered more frequently with TandemHeart PVAD support.[26] In another retrospective study, TandemHeart PVAD was used in 117 patients (80 ischemic cardiomyopathy, 37 nonischemic cardiomyopathy) with SRCS and was associated with marked improvement in hemodynamics (increased mean arterial pressure [MAP], mixed venous oxygenation saturation, and urine output along with decreased pulmonary capillary wedge pressure) and end-organ perfusion (decreased lactic acid and creatinine). The overall 30-day and 6-month mortality rates in this cohort were 40.2% and 45.3%, respectively.[27]

The TandemHeart PVAD has also been validated in smaller series as a successful bridge-to-transplant,[28] bridge-to-bridge,[29] bridge-to-decision,[30] and bridge-to-recovery[31] device. In addition, recent single-center studies suggest that the TandemHeart PVAD is effective when used for circulatory support for high-risk PCI, with an acceptably low rate of device-related complications.[32,33]

Impella Recover 2.5 PVAD and Impellac VAD

The ImpellaRecover 2.5 PVAD (Abiomed Inc) is FDA-approved for up to 6 hours of partial circulatory support and is capable of augmenting CO by 2.5 L/min. The ISAR-SHOCK trial, in patients with LV failure after AMI, showed the Impella Recover 2.5 PVAD had significantly greater augmentation of MAP and cardiac index with rapid decrease in serum lactate levels after 30 minutes of support, compared with patients supported by IABP. However, overall 30-day mortality was 46% in both groups. A higher incidence of hemolysis in patients treated with Impella PVAD support was also noted.[34] Recent data from the EUROSHOCK registry on the use of the Impella 2.5 PVAD in patients with cardiogenic shock suggested improvement in 48-hour serum lactate levels and improved end-organ perfusion. However, the 30-day rate of mortality remained high (64.2%).[35]

More recent data by Engstrom and colleagues[36] suggests that the Impella Recover 5.0 device may be more appropriate than the Impella Recover 2.5 PVAD for patients with SRCS after STEMI if a surgical team is available. They also recommended using the Impella 2.5 system as a bridge to Impella 5.0 system in patients unable to get an Impella 5.0 system initially.

The IMPRESS in STEMI trial, which aimed at evaluating the mechanical support of IABP versus IMPELLA 2.5 in patients with STEMI with signs of preshock, was recently stopped because of low inclusion rate.[37] In addition, the RECOVER II trial, which aimed at comparing IABP support versus Impella 2.5 in hemodynamically unstable STEMI patients, was also stopped due to insufficient enrollment.[38]

Impellac VAD is the most recently developed Impella recover system, capable of generating up to 4 L/min of CO. It can be implanted percutaneously and was recently used successfully for hemodynamic support in an 85-year-old patient with complex coronary artery disease, decreased LV ejection fraction, and prior MI. The IMPRESS in Severe Shock Trial, which aims to evaluate the efficacy of Impellac VAD in patients with cardiogenic shock, is currently enrolling patients and will provide more insight into the use of PVADs for LVCS.[39]

The PROTECT I trial evaluated the Impella 2.5 for hemodynamic support during high-risk PCI. All patients underwent successful device implantation, with cases of procedure-related hemodynamic compromise or limb ischemia, a 10% incidence of hemolysis, and a 30-day MACE rate of 20%.[40] The follow-up, PROTECT II trial, was a randomized controlled trial done in patients with complex 3-vessel disease or unprotected left main coronary artery disease and severely depressed LV systolic function, with patients randomized to IABP or Impella 2.5 support during nonemergent high-risk PCI. Although the Impella 2.5 provided superior hemodynamic support, the rates of 30-day MACE were not statistically different and the trial was stopped by DSMB. However, there was a strong trend toward a decrease in 90-day MACE in the Impella 2.5 group.[41]

Additional data from 144 patients in the Europella Registry, all of whom underwent Impella Recover 2.5 PVAD-assisted high-risk PCI, demonstrated 30-day mortality of 5.5% and a low incidence of adverse events.[42] The USpella is the largest registry of multicenter, real-world high-risk PCI with Impella 2.5 used in 175 patients. It showed a low 30-day MACE rate of 8% with a 0.9% revascularization rate.[43] In addition, Impella 2.5 has also been used for high-risk/unstable ventricular tachycardia ablation.[52]

Percutaneous ECMO

ECMO is gaining favor for LVCS because of improved cannulae, oxygenators, as well as overall device miniaturization (**Fig. 3**). ECMO offers a

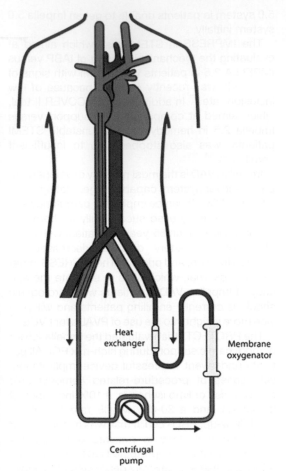

Fig. 3. A percutaneous veno-arterial access. The venous access is connected to an extracorporeal membrane oxygenation (ECMO) system with an integrated centrifugal pump and membrane oxygenator (artificial lung) and connected to the arterial inflow access. (*From* Ouweneel DM, Henriques JP. Percutaneous cardiac support devices for cardiogenic shock: current indications and recommendations. Heart 2012;98(16): 1246–54; with permission.)

rapid method of percutaneous cardiopulmonary support without the need for transseptal puncture or transfer to a catheterization laboratory and is increasingly being used with success in tertiary care centers as a means to bridge to permanent assist device implantation or transplantation. ECMO has been used for short-term cardiopulmonary support in patients with postcardiotomy CS,[44] as a bridge-to-recovery in patients with fulminant myocarditis,[45] and has been shown to improve 30-day outcomes when used for hemodynamic support during primary PCI in patients presenting with STEMI and profound CS.[46]

Newer versions of ECMO are smaller and are now being increasingly used as a Mobile Remote Cardiac Assist unit in remote centers in patients with SRCS before transfer to tertiary centers. The CARDIOHELP system (Maquet AG, Hirrlingen, Germany) is a hand-held mini-ECMO system that has been FDA approved as a bridge to recovery in out-of-hospital patients with SRCS.[47] Similarly, the LIFEBRIDGE-B2T (Medizintechnik AG, Ampfing, Germany) system is a portable cardiopulmonary bypass system capable of providing 3 to 4 L/min of cardiac support, which is FDA approved for 6 hours of support and has been used to support high-risk PCI in a patient with CS[48] as well as pulmonary embolectomy in a patient with cardiovascular collapse.[49]

New PVADs for LV Shock

Several new PVADs are now being tested for hemodynamic support of patients in CS. New PVADs include the Reitan Catheter Pump (Kiwimed, London, UK) as well as the the iVAC 3L PVAD (PulseCath BV, Amsterdam, Netherlands). The Reitan catheter pump is a catheter-mounted foldable propeller capable of providing up to 5 L/min of circulatory support. It is deployed in the descending aorta and reduces afterload by creating a negative pressure gradient. The iVAC 3L PVAD (PulseCath BV) is a 17-F or 21-F catheter-based system capable of providing pulsatile flow of 2 to 3 L/min from the LV into the ascending aorta. Studies demonstrating the hemodynamic effects of these devices in humans are awaited.

PVADS: IMPORTANT CLINICAL CONSIDERATIONS
Patient Stabilization and Transfer

Partnerships should be set up between smaller peripheral hospitals and central hospitals capable of PVAD-mediated circulatory support and high-risk interventions. Patients presenting to the peripheral hospitals should be stabilized with securing the airway, mechanical ventilation, vasopressor/inotrope initiation, and placement of an IABP as well as primary PCI. If the patient's clinical condition further deteriorates, they should be transferred rapidly to the central hospital before development of refractory cardiogenic shock. At these central hospitals, similar to STEMI activation, a well-defined PVAD team needs to be activated before patient arrival. This team would consist of physicians, nurses, catheterization laboratory technicians, and circulatory support technicians with easy access to prepackaged PVAD kits containing all the materials required for PVAD insertion.

Appropriate Patient Selection

The goal of PVAD support initiation is to improve survival, rather than prolong the process of dying, and this should guide the selection of candidates.[50] Therefore, after evaluation by a multidisciplinary team including the patient's family and treating physician, if there is no foreseeable exit strategy for PVAD removal (ie, bridge-to-revascularization, bridge-to-recovery, bridge-to-bridge [surgical LVAD], bridge-to-transplant, or bridge-to-decision [additional time required to assess likelihood of recovery]), PVAD therapy should be withheld. In this circumstance, end-of-life issues and palliative care should be addressed.

Appropriate Device Selection

Several factors govern the choice of a particular PVAD in each patient. The most important factors are the degree of mechanical support needed to restore perfusion and the adequacy of oxygenation. Right ventricular (RV) function plays a key role in determining the amount of mechanical support needed. RV dysfunction would necessitate urgent correction of acidosis, consideration of pharmacologic support (ie, pulmonary vasodilators and/or inotropes), and possibly mechanical support targeted at unloading the RV (eg, percutaneous RV assist device, percutaneous biventricular assist device, or veno-arterial ECMO). Other factors for PVAD selection include end-organ dysfunction and comorbidities (eg, peripheral vascular disease). In patients requiring mechanical support for a prolonged period, biventricular failure, those with severe peripheral arterial disease, or postcardiotomy CS, surgically implanted temporary VAD insertion is preferred. **Fig. 4** depicts a suggested approach to PVAD selection for acute cardiopulmonary failure.

Optimal Timing of Implantation

Initiation of vasopressor and/or inotropic support in CS achieves short-term hemodynamic improvement while simultaneously increasing the oxygen demand and ATP consumption in the failing myocardium, which leads to a profound supply-demand mismatch propagating a vicious cycle. Thus, there is a narrow window of opportunity whereby early institution of mechanical circulatory support via IABP and/or PVADs could break the cycle instead of continued escalation of medical therapy.

Hemodynamic Goals and PVAD Weaning

Efforts should be made to maintain physiologic parameters (mean arterial pressure >60 mm Hg and a mixed venous oxygen saturation of >70%) during PVAD support. PVAD weaning, done by gradually decreasing PVAD speed/flow and gradually reloading the ventricle, should be attempted in patients who demonstrate hemodynamic stability (including minimal/no pressor requirement) and improved end-organ function. Patients failing to recover should be transitioned to a long-term surgical VAD or transplantation.

Potential Complications

PVAD support is associated with several complications. Limb ischemia is more likely in the setting of severe peripheral vascular disease with PVADs requiring large-bore access. Therefore, review of the arterial anatomy is critical during consideration of cannula size and antegrade perfusion catheter placement may be used to prevent subclinical

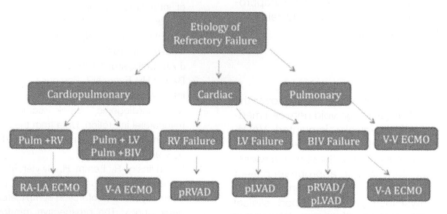

Fig. 4. Proposed strategy for PVAD selection in acute cardiopulmonary failure. BIV, Biventricular; pLVAD, percutaneous left ventricular assist device; pRVAD, percutaneous right ventricular assist device; RA-LA, Right atrial-left atrial; RV, right ventricle; V-A, Veno-arterial; V-V ECMO, Veno-venous extra corporeal membrane oxygenation.

limb ischemia and/or reperfusion injury on device removal. Another complication associated with PVAD support is hemolysis, seen more frequently with high-turbulence microaxial devices like the Impella Recover 2.5 PVAD. Thrombotic complications such as strokes and emboli are decreased by continuous anticoagulation with intravenous heparin drip to maintain an activated clotting time greater than 300 seconds. In addition, PVAD pump speeds should be decreased to allow intermittent opening of the aortic valve to avoid stagnation of blood in the aortic root and thrombus formation.[51] Increased pump speeds also lead to over-decompression of the LV, which can cause suction of the interventricular septum toward the PVAD inlet cannula, obstructing inlet flow and potentially precipitating VT or RV failure by septal shift. Optimal pump speeds for adequate unloading while avoiding complications associated with over-decompression should be established with frequent speed-change echocardiograms in all patients.

Future Directions of PVAD Research

Although multiple studies have shown significant improvement in hemodynamic parameters and end-organ function in patients with LVCS, it has been difficult to demonstrate a mortality benefit with PVADs in randomized trials. A potential cause for this is the ethical dilemma of randomizing critically ill patients to IABP, who otherwise meet criteria (as defined by FDA 510k documents) for PVADs. It is important to realize that PVAD implantation is not a definitive therapy by itself in most cases (except myocarditis) and outcomes likely depend on the exit strategy used (high-risk PCI/valve repair/bridge to transplant/bridge to LVAD) while on PVAD support. Other challenges currently associated with PVAD research include inappropriate patient and device selection and relatively late initiation of PVAD support.

SUMMARY

PVADs for LVCS have developed rapidly over the last decade and bridge a huge void between medical therapies and surgically implanted VADs. There is, however, a lack of randomized trial data evaluating the effectiveness of these new devices. Areas of further study include appropriate patient and device selection, timing of implantation and explanation, physiologic goals of support, clinical outcomes, and cost-effectiveness. While this occurs, the development of novel and versatile PVAD technologies continues.

REFERENCES

1. Levine GN, Bates ER, Blankenship JC, et al. 2011 ACCF/AHA/SCAI guideline for percutaneous coronary intervention: a report of the American College of Cardiology Foundation/American Heart Association task force on practice guidelines and the Society for Cardiovascular Angiography and Interventions. Circulation 2011;124:e574–651.

2. Kar B, Basra SS, Shah NR, et al. Percutaneous circulatory support in cardiogenic shock: Interventional bridge to recovery. Circulation 2012;125:1809–17.

3. Babaev A, Frederick PD, Pasta DJ, et al. Trends in management and outcomes of patients with acute myocardial infarction complicated by cardiogenic shock. JAMA 2005;294:448–54.

4. Hasdai D, Harrington RA, Hochman JS, et al. Platelet glycoprotein IIb/IIIa blockade and outcome of cardiogenic shock complicating acute coronary syndromes without persistent st-segment elevation. J Am Coll Cardiol 2000;36:685–92.

5. Hochman JS, Sleeper LA, Webb JG, et al. Early revascularization in acute myocardial infarction complicated by cardiogenic shock. Shock investigators. Should we emergently revascularize occluded coronaries for cardiogenic shock. N Engl J Med 1999;341:625–34.

6. Scheidt S, Wilner G, Mueller H, et al. Intra-aortic balloon counterpulsation in cardiogenic shock. Report of a co-operative clinical trial. N Engl J Med 1973;288:979–84.

7. Sanborn TA, Sleeper LA, Bates ER, et al. Impact of thrombolysis, intra-aortic balloon pump counterpulsation, and their combination in cardiogenic shock complicating acute myocardial infarction: A report from the Shock Trial Registry. Should we emergently revascularize occluded coronaries for cardiogenic shock? J Am Coll Cardiol 2000;36:1123–9.

8. Anderson RD, Ohman EM, Holmes DR Jr, et al. Use of intraaortic balloon counterpulsation in patients presenting with cardiogenic shock: observations from the gusto-i study. Global utilization of streptokinase and tpa for occluded coronary arteries. J Am Coll Cardiol 1997;30:708–15.

9. Barron HV, Every NR, Parsons LS, et al. The use of intra-aortic balloon counterpulsation in patients with cardiogenic shock complicating acute myocardial infarction: Data from the national registry of myocardial infarction 2. Am Heart J 2001;141:933–9.

10. Prondzinsky R, Lemm H, Swyter M, et al. Intra-aortic balloon counterpulsation in patients with acute myocardial infarction complicated by cardiogenic shock: The prospective, randomized IABP shock trial for attenuation of multiorgan dysfunction syndrome. Crit Care Med 2010;38:152–60.

11. Unverzagt S, Machemer MT, Solms A, et al. Intra-aortic balloon pump counterpulsation (IABP) for myocardial infarction complicated by cardiogenic shock. Cochrane Database Syst Rev 2011;(7):CD007398.

12. Sjauw KD, Engstrom AE, Vis MM, et al. A systematic review and meta-analysis of intra-aortic balloon pump therapy in ST-elevation myocardial infarction: Should we change the guidelines? Eur Heart J 2009; 30:459–68.

13. Perera D, Stables R, Thomas M, et al. Elective intra-aortic balloon counterpulsation during high-risk percutaneous coronary intervention: a randomized controlled trial. JAMA 2010;304:867–74.

14. Patel MR, Smalling RW, Thiele H, et al. Intra-aortic balloon counterpulsation and infarct size in patients with acute anterior myocardial infarction without shock: the crisp AMI randomized trial. JAMA 2011;306:1329–37.

15. Thiele H, Zeymer U, Neumann FJ, et al. Intraaortic balloon support for myocardial infarction with cardiogenic shock. N Engl J Med 2012;367:1287–96.

16. Akay MH, Gregoric ID, Radovancevic R, et al. Timely use of a centrimag heart assist device improves survival in postcardiotomy cardiogenic shock. J Cardiovasc Surg 2011;26:548–52.

17. John R, Long JW, Massey HT, et al. Outcomes of a multicenter trial of the levitronix centrimag ventricular assist system for short-term circulatory support. J Thorac Cardiovasc Surg 2011;141:932–9.

18. Thomas HL, Dronavalli VB, Parameshwar J, et al. Incidence and outcome of levitronix centrimag support as rescue therapy for early cardiac allograft failure: a united kingdom national study. Eur J Cardiothorac Surg 2011;40(6):1348–54.

19. Aziz TA, Singh G, Popjes E, et al. Initial experience with centrimag extracorporal membrane oxygenation for support of critically ill patients with refractory cardiogenic shock. J Heart Lung Transplant 2010;29:66–71.

20. LaRocca GM, Shimbo D, Rodriguez CJ, et al. The Impella Recover LP 5.0 left ventricular assist device: a bridge to coronary artery bypass grafting and cardiac transplantation. J Am Soc Echocardiogr 2006;19(468):e465–7.

21. Samoukovic G, Rosu C, Giannetti N, et al. The Impella LP 5.0 as a bridge to long-term circulatory support. Interact Cardiovasc Thorac Surg 2009;8: 682–3.

22. Samoukovic G, Al-Atassi T, Rosu C, et al. Successful treatment of heart failure due to acute transplant rejection with the Impella LP 5.0. Ann Thorac Surg 2009;88:271–3.

23. Andrade JG, Al-Saloos H, Jeewa A, et al. Facilitated cardiac recovery in fulminant myocarditis: pediatric use of the Impella LP 5.0 pump. J Heart Lung Transplant 2010;29:96–7.

24. Fonger JD, Zhou Y, Matsuura H, et al. Enhanced preservation of acutely ischemic myocardium with transseptal left ventricular assist. Ann Thorac Surg 1994;57:570–5.

25. Burkhoff D, Cohen H, Brunckhorst C, et al. A randomized multicenter clinical study to evaluate the safety and efficacy of the Tandemheart percutaneous ventricular assist device versus conventional therapy with intraaortic balloon pumping for treatment of cardiogenic shock. Am Heart J 2006; 152:469.e1–8.

26. Thiele H, Sick P, Boudriot E, et al. Randomized comparison of intra-aortic balloon support with a percutaneous left ventricular assist device in patients with revascularized acute myocardial infarction complicated by cardiogenic shock. Eur Heart J 2005;26: 1276–83.

27. Kar B, Gregoric ID, Basra SS, et al. The percutaneous ventricular assist device in severe refractory cardiogenic shock. J Am Coll Cardiol 2011;57: 688–96.

28. Bruckner BA, Jacob LP, Gregoric ID, et al. Clinical experience with the Tandemheart percutaneous ventricular assist device as a bridge to cardiac transplantation. Tex Heart Inst J 2008;35:447–50.

29. Gregoric ID, Jacob LP, La Francesca S, et al. The Tandemheart as a bridge to a long-term axial-flow left ventricular assist device (bridge to bridge). Tex Heart Inst J 2008;35:125–9.

30. Brinkman WT, Rosenthal JE, Eichhorn E, et al. Role of a percutaneous ventricular assist device in decision making for a cardiac transplant program. Ann Thorac Surg 2009;88:1462–6.

31. Chandra D, Kar B, Idelchik G, et al. Usefulness of percutaneous left ventricular assist device as a bridge to recovery from myocarditis. Am J Cardiol 2007;99:1755–6.

32. Kar B, Forrester M, Gemmato C, et al. Use of the Tandemheart percutaneous ventricular assist device to support patients undergoing high-risk percutaneous coronary intervention. J Invasive Cardiol 2006;18:93–6.

33. Vranckx P, Meliga E, De Jaegere PP, et al. The Tandemheart, percutaneous transseptal left ventricular assist device: a safeguard in high-risk percutaneous coronary interventions. The six-year rotterdam experience. EuroIntervention 2008;4: 331–7.

34. Seyfarth M, Sibbing D, Bauer I, et al. A randomized clinical trial to evaluate the safety and efficacy of a percutaneous left ventricular assist device versus intra-aortic balloon pumping for treatment of cardiogenic shock caused by myocardial infarction. J Am Coll Cardiol 2008;52:1584–8.

35. Lauten A, Engstrom AE, Jung C, et al. Percutaneous left-ventricular support with the impella-2.5-assist device in acute cardiogenic shock: results

of the impella-euroshock-registry. Circ Heart Fail 2013;6:23–30.

36. Engstrom AE, Cocchieri R, Driessen AH, et al. The Impella 2.5 and 5.0 devices for ST-elevation myocardial infarction patients presenting with severe and profound cardiogenic shock: the academic medical center intensive care unit experience. Crit Care Med 2011;39(9):2072–9.

37. Impress in STEMI trial. Available at: http://www.trialregister.nl/trialreg/admin/rctview.asp?tc=1079.

38. Recover trial I impella Recover LP/LD 5.0 support system safety and feasibility study.

39. Impress in severe shock. Available at: http://www.trialregister.nl/trialreg/admin/rctview.asp?TC=3450.

40. Dixon SR, Henriques JP, Mauri L, et al. A prospective feasibility trial investigating the use of the Impella 2.5 system in patients undergoing high-risk percutaneous coronary intervention (the protect I trial): initial U.S. experience. JACC Cardiovasc Interv 2009;2:91–6.

41. O'Neill WW, Kleiman NS, Moses J, et al. A prospective, randomized clinical trial of hemodynamic support with Impella 2.5 versus intra-aortic balloon pump in patients undergoing high-risk percutaneous coronary intervention: the PROTECT II study. Circulation 2012;126:1717–27.

42. Sjauw KD, Konorza T, Erbel R, et al. Supported high-risk percutaneous coronary intervention with the Impella 2.5 device the Europella registry. J Am Coll Cardiol 2009;54:2430–4.

43. Maini B, Naidu SS, Mulukutla S, et al. Real-world use of the Impella 2.5 circulatory support system in complex high-risk percutaneous coronary intervention: the Uspella registry. Catheter Cardiovasc Interv 2012;80:717–25.

44. Doll N, Kiaii B, Borger M, et al. Five-year results of 219 consecutive patients treated with extracorporeal membrane oxygenation for refractory postoperative cardiogenic shock. Ann Thorac Surg 2004;77:151–7 [discussion: 157].

45. Asaumi Y, Yasuda S, Morii I, et al. Favourable clinical outcome in patients with cardiogenic shock due to fulminant myocarditis supported by percutaneous extracorporeal membrane oxygenation. Eur Heart J 2005;26:2185–92.

46. Sheu JJ, Tsai TH, Lee FY, et al. Early extracorporeal membrane oxygenator-assisted primary percutaneous coronary intervention improved 30-day clinical outcomes in patients with st-segment elevation myocardial infarction complicated with profound cardiogenic shock. Crit Care Med 2010;38:1810–7.

47. Arlt M, Philipp A, Voelkel S, et al. Hand-held minimised extracorporeal membrane oxygenation: a new bridge to recovery in patients with out-of-centre cardiogenic shock. Eur J Cardiothorac Surg 2011;40(3):689–94.

48. Jung C, Schlosser M, Figulla HR, et al. Providing macro- and microcirculatory support with the life-bridge system during high-risk PCI in cardiogenic shock. Heart Lung Circ 2009;18:296–8.

49. Conzelmann LO, Mehlhorn U, Weigang E, et al. Successful management of fulminant pulmonary embolism using a novel portable extracorporeal life support system. Ann Thorac Surg 2011;91:1265–7.

50. Tallaj JA, Cadeiras M. Mechanical rescue of the heart in shock. J Am Coll Cardiol 2011;57:697–9.

51. Demirozu ZT, Ho J, Bogaev RC, et al. Thrombotic occlusion of an aortic-root xenograft during left ventricular assistance. Tex Heart Inst J 2011;38:66–7.

52. Abuissa H, Roshan J, Lim B, et al. Use of the Impella microaxial blood pump for ablation of hemodynamically unstable ventricular tachycardia. J Cardiovasc Electrophysiol 2010;21(4):458–61.

Percutaneous Assist Devices for Infarct Size Reduction

Hammad Saudye, MD, Kirk N. Garratt, MSc, MD*

KEYWORDS

- Percutaneous assist devices • Infarct size reduction • Acute myocardial infarction
- Myocardial salvage

KEY POINTS

- A percutaneous left ventricular (LV) assist device could improve myocyte salvage during acute myocardial infarction (AMI) therapy if it is able to reduce myocardial oxygen demand, wall tension, and LV stroke work substantially.
- An ideal percutaneous LV assist device should be readily manageable by a catheterization laboratory team, reduce LV stroke work by more than 50%, and sustain adequate systemic perfusion to maintain organ viability even when intrinsic cardiac function is minimal, in addition to reducing infarct size.
- Of the 3 devices widely available in North America, only the intra-aortic balloon pump has been adequately tested in human studies to determine its ability to reduce final infarct size; it was found to provide insufficient LV unloading to achieve this goal.
- Both the Impella (Abiomed, Danvers, MA) and the TandemHeart (CardiacAssist Inc, Pittsburgh, PA) are in the early phases of human subject clinical studies aimed at determining if they can interfere with lethal reperfusion injury and programmed cell death following AMI. Both devices are being assessed for feasibility of use in the setting of AMI; if feasibility studies are successful, pivotal efficacy trials are expected to follow.

MYOCARDIAL RESPONSE TO ISCHEMIC INJURY

The myocardial response to ischemia is well documented. Within seconds of ischemia, preceding any myocardial necrosis, regional functional abnormality proceeds through a process of dyssynchrony, hypokinesis, akinesis, and paradoxic systolic expansion.[1] The first detectable change in response to hypoxia is a lengthening of the muscle fibers during isovolumic contraction and relaxation phases. This lengthening results in hypoxic tissue stretching while normal tissue contracts in systole, a paradoxic motion. Lengthening is also seen in diastole with a change in regional diastolic segment length of 5% to 20%. Systolic function is not compromised during initial hypoxia, but myocytes lose the ability to contract as ischemia progresses, resulting in a reduction in force generation and regional hypokinesis that progresses to akinesis and passive diastolic stretching of the ischemic tissue by adjacent normal myocardium. Once this area is elongated, normal myocardium continues to contract, pulling on the myocardium and causing paradoxic expansion of the infarct zone during systole.

On a hemodynamic level, this is reflected by an early increase in left ventricular end-diastolic pressure (LVEDP) as well as depression in systolic function. Varying degrees of diastolic function have shown to be prognostic in the setting of acute myocardial infarction (AMI). Restrictive filling pattern is associated with heart failure after MI[2] and is an independent predictor of mortality after AMI regardless of LVEF, end-systolic volume index,

Department of Cardiology, Northshore-LIJ/Lenox Hill Hospital, New York, NY 10075, USA
* Corresponding author. 130 East 77th Street, 9th Floor, New York, NY 10075.
E-mail address: KGarratt@NSHS.edu

Intervent Cardiol Clin 2 (2013) 469–484
http://dx.doi.org/10.1016/j.iccl.2013.04.003
2211-7458/13/$ – see front matter © 2013 Elsevier Inc. All rights reserved.

and Killip class.[3] Lesser diastolic dysfunction, a pseudonormal pattern with elevated filling pressures based on E/e' measurements, has been related to adverse outcomes following AMI.[4] It has been shown that mitral deceleration time, systolic wall motion index, and other measures are related to survival in a graded fashion (**Fig. 1**).[5]

Cardiac output declines as myocardial contractility decreases, affecting end organ perfusion and coronary blood flow, thereby propagating ischemia. As myofibril shortening ceases and passive stretching ensues, the end-systolic volume increases. Once myocardium dilates beyond the ability of the myocytes to restore shape, the infarct zone thins, the area of injury stretches further, and further LV dilatation takes place. Dilatation results in increased wall tension and further oxygen demand for remaining viable myocytes. Contractility of the LV is impaired not just because of ischemia but also because of deranged systolic and diastolic dimensions. Secondary changes also occur in the left atrium; the composite of these changes has been linked to increased rates of death and hospitalization for heart failure after AMI.[6]

Under normal conditions, the heart extracts more oxygen from blood than any other organ in the body. Typical arterial oxygen content is 20 mL of oxygen per 100 mL of blood; the kidneys extract 3 to 5 mL of blood, and the heart extracts approximately 10 to 12 mL O_2/100 mL of blood.[7] Because the myocardium relies almost completely on aerobic metabolism, the supply of oxygen to the myocardium is determined by oxygen carrying capacity and coronary blood flow.[8] Oxygen carrying capacity is only compromised in situations of carbon monoxide poisoning, severe hypoxia, or significant anemia. Coronary blood flow, however, is much more variable. It is directly related to the pressure gradient across the myocardial

capillary bed and inversely related to the resistance in flow. The driving force is essentially diastolic blood pressure minus right atrial pressure. Resistance to flow is multifactorial and is determined by metabolic needs (maintaining a set point concentration of metabolites like adenosine)[9]; autoregulation[10] (to maintain coronary perfusion pressure between 60–160 mm Hg); external compressive forces[11] (systolic compression and twist on the coronaries, accounting for almost 50% of the resistance); diastolic interval (duration of flow to the subendocardium); humoral control (vasoactive amines such as angiotensin 2 acting on endothelial cells); and neural control[12] (with alpha adrenergic stimulation inducing coronary constriction and beta adrenergic and parasympathetic stimulation inducing vasodilatation.) On the other side of the equation, oxygen demand is related to heart rate, contractility, and wall tension.[13] Because wall tension is directly related to pressure and radius and inversely related to wall thickness (law of Laplace), it is easy to understand how elevated LVEDP and LV end-diastolic volume (LVEDV) can impact the oxygen demand. Furthermore, as stroke volume decreases, tachycardia ensues to compensate for the decline in cardiac output, creating additional increases in oxygen demand. Thus, the balance between oxygen supply and oxygen demand is badly disrupted during periods of severe ischemic stress (**Fig. 2**).

Yellon and Hausenloy[14] estimate that acute coronary occlusion puts about 70% of heart tissue perfused by the involved artery at risk of ischemic death; about 30% of heart tissue will survive, even if the vessel is left occluded, because of endogenous protective mechanisms, particularly recruitment of collateral blood flow. With acute reperfusion, much of the threatened tissue is salvaged. The degree of tissue salvage

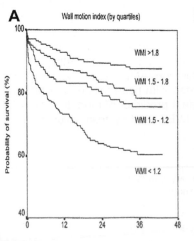
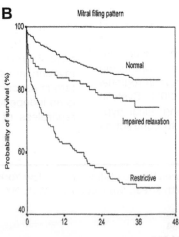

Fig. 1. Influence of MI on survival after AMI. (*A*) Survival as a function of echocardiographic LV wall motion index (WMI) after AMI. (*B*) Survival as a function of echocardiographic mitral valve filling patterns after AMI. (*From* Møller JE, Egstrup K, Køber L, et al. Prognostic importance of systolic and diastolic function after acute myocardial infarction. Am Heart J 2003;145: 147–53; with permission.)

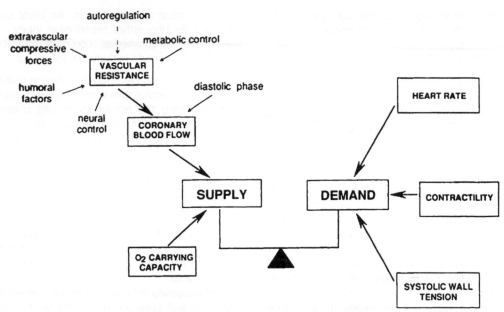

Fig. 2. Factors influencing the supply and demand for oxygen within myocytes. (*From* Ardehali A, Ports TA. Myocardial oxygen supply and demand. Chest 1990;98:699–705; with permission.)

is time dependent. Even with early reperfusion, some permanent tissue injury may occur; some tissue undergoes ischemic necrosis promptly, but much of the threatened, viable tissue progresses to death hours to days later. The mechanisms underlying this phenomenon are highly complex and incompletely understood, but sufficient progress has been made to offer potential therapeutic options to enhance myocardial salvage following AMI[15]; herein lays opportunities for additional myocardial salvage.

OPPORTUNITIES FOR ADDITIONAL MYOCARDIAL SALVAGE

A recent study of patients with AMI with proximal left anterior decending (LAD) occlusions that were relieved with primary angioplasty within 90 minutes of presentation showed myocardial salvage of only 35% of the area at risk, as measured with cardiac magnetic resonance imaging (MRI).[16] Although opening an occluded vessel restores aerobic metabolism and function to some myocytes, epicardial flow restoration does not necessarily equate to microvascular flow. Approximately 6% of myocardium may show evidence of microvascular obstruction even after successful, early reperfusion.[2] But beyond microvascular obstruction, mechanisms are activated that lead to apoptosis or programed cell death. This field is very complex and growing quickly. Evidence now exists for many molecular mediators of death signaling, with at

least 2 separate apoptotic pathways[17]: one (sometimes called the intrinsic pathway) related to the activity of regulator proteins first described as having an important role in certain types of lymphomas (B-cell lymphoma 2, or Bcl-2, proteins) and another (sometimes called the *extrinsic pathway*) involving the FAS receptor, a membrane-bound member of the tumor-necrosis factor superfamily of receptors that is known to form a death-inducing signaling complex when it interacts with an appropriate ligand.[17–19] As much as 50% of the final infarct size may be attributable to apoptosis or other death signal-mediated consequences of reperfusion injury.[14] Countering these death pathways are salvage pathways. Many seem to exist, but perhaps the best studied is the reperfusion injury signaling kinase (RISK) pathway.[20,21] Briefly, this system of enzymes protects against lethal reperfusion-induced injury if activated within the first few minutes of reperfusion. The exact mechanisms are not known, but a principal target of this system is the permeability-transition pore of mitochondria.[22] Lethal ischemic injury leads to the opening of this pore, which becomes irreversible at a certain point. The RISK pathway prevents the permeability-transition pore from reaching this critical opening size and leads to closure of the pore, restoring normality and preventing cell death. The RISK pathway also restores and maintains the integrity of certain ion-regulating membrane channels (especially the K_{ATP} channel) that are integral to cell membrane integrity and normal energetics.[23]

Influencing death signaling and salvage systems would provide an opportunity to control lethal reperfusion injury.

Many pharmacologic therapies have been studied in efforts to reduce final infarct size, but almost all have failed. Cyclosporine, thought to have a role in regulation of the permeability transition pore, was associated with a smaller infarct size when administered to a small number of patients.[15] Adenosine infusion was associated with a reduction in mean infarct size among patients with anterior wall AMIs,[24] with the greatest impact seen among those patients who presented with a short ischemic time[25]; adenosine may be most likely to be helpful because it is known to interfere with more than one of the mechanisms postulated to contribute to reperfusion injury.[26] Beyond these two compounds, 20 years of pharmacologic intervention studies have yielded little to benefit patients with AMI.

The best-established mechanical therapy to enhance myocyte salvage is the decompression of LV pressures. In the setting of myocardial ischemia during cardiac surgeries, LV decompression has been used for more than 3 decades to limit ischemic injury.[27,28] Animal research provides convincing evidence that unloading of LV pressure reduces final myocardial infarct size; the magnitude of benefit is linked to the degree of LV unloading. Animal studies suggest that for LV unloading to effect significant injury reductions, the LV must be relieved of more than 50% of its energy requirement.[27,28] This task is easily achievable during cardiac surgery when open cardiopulmonary bypass can be used to completely unload the heart; the task is more difficult for percutaneous devices. The mechanistic goal of pressure relief is to reduce energy requirements through substantial reduction in cardiac work. Of course, critical organ

perfusion must be maintained. An ideal device, then, for limiting lethal reperfusion injury in the setting of percutaneous coronary intervention (PCI) for AMI should include the following:

1. It should be simple enough in design that interventional cardiologists can place it percutaneously using the resources usually present in the cardiac catheterization laboratory.
2. It should relieve the LV pressure and volume as completely as possible to permit complete LV rest.
3. It should simultaneously provide perfusion support that is adequate to meet the metabolic demands of critical organs.

To assess the potential utility of devices for limiting infarct size, we must consider the ability of any candidate device to lower LV energy requirements.

Cardiac power output (in joules) is defined as the mean arterial pressure multiplied by the cardiac output and divided by 451 (CPO = [MAP × CO]/451), where *CPO* is cardiac power output, *MAP* is mean arterial pressure, and *CO* is cardiac output. It represents not only the mechanical work required to pump blood out of the ventricle but also the potential energy stored in the Frank-Starling forces at rest; this concept is best represented in pressure-volume loops (**Fig. 3**). The focus when reviewing pressure-volume loops is typically on the area bounded by the loop because this area reflects cardiac work done during a single cardiac systolic-diastolic cycle and provides important information about stroke volume and cardiac output. Oxygen consumption correlates directly with the area enclosed by the pressure-volume loop,[28] so cardiac power correlates with cardiac oxygen demand. However, this area does not account for all oxygen demand; energy

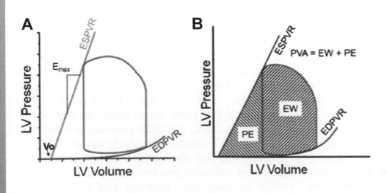

Fig. 3. Relationship between LV pressure, LV volume, and LV energy requirements. (*A*) Pressure-volume loop relationship to maximal end-diastolic pressure and theoretical LV volume corresponding to minimal transmural stress. (*B*) Determination of total energy requirement for the LV. EDPVR, end-diastolic pressure-volume relationship; E_{max}, slope of line passing from V_0 to end-systolic pressure-volume point; ESPVR, end-systolic pressure-volume relationship; EW, external work (related to kinetic energy requirement of contractility); PE, potential energy (related to ventricular wall stress during diastole); V_0, unstressed LV volume. (*From* Kawashima D, Gojo S, Nishimura T, et al. Impella provides more ventricular unloading in heart failure than extracorporeal membrane oxygenation. ASAIO J 2011;57:169–76; with permission.)

is required to maintain the LV under a passive load when muscle is not actively contracting. This static phase energy requirement is sometimes called the *potential energy requirement* of the LV. For the purposes of reducing final infarct size, both the active (kinetic) energy of contractility and the static (potential) energy of load maintenance must be addressed. As shown in **Fig. 4**, the active energy requirement generated by one cardiac cycle approaches 100 cJ. The energy requirement related to maintenance of the basal resting state is about one-third the active energy requirement. Combining both of these figures accounts for the total LV energy requirement over a single cardiac cycle; this total energy requirement is reflected graphically by the area bounded by the total pressure-volume area. Importantly, myocardial potential energy is related to wall tension; maximal wall tension develops at end diastole, so mechanical interventions most likely to improve myocardial salvage should reduce the end-diastolic pressure-volume value as well as the systolic pressure-volume peak value.

Three percutaneous devices have been suggested for use in AMI to reduce infarct size; to some degree, all have been applied in clinical practice: (1) intra-aortic balloon counterpulsation pump (IABP) devices, (2) the Impella device (Abiomed, Danvers, MA), and (3) the TandemHeart device (CardiacAssist Inc, Pittsburgh, PA). The surgical extracorporeal membrane oxygenator perfusion system (ECMO) is also used to support patients with critical loss of cardiac function, particularly those with biventricular failure; but this system has not been studied as a means of improving myocardial salvage during AMI.

IABP

IABP devices have been deployed widely for about 40 years. They have been used chiefly to support failing hearts or to provide additional support during angioplasty procedures predicted to have higher risk of hemodynamic compromise.[29] Recently, IABP placement for the purposes of reducing final infarct size has been explored. The logic of this approach has been challenged because an IABP has limited ability to effect LV unloading.[30] In patients with AMI complicated by cardiogenic shock, for example, differences in pressure-volume loops with and without IABP support may be trivial (**Fig. 5**). Still the device is capable of reducing LV cardiac work during the earliest part of systole and is familiar and widely available, so it is of interest to clinicians.

Some animal studies suggested that LV unloading with IABP could be substantial and beneficial. Fonger and colleagues[27] observed a marked reduction in LVEDP as a result of IABP support in anesthetized pigs subjected to balloon occlusion of coronary arteries. Investigators at the University of Athens in Greece found smaller final infarcts, as a percentage of the area at risk, when IABP assistance was used for 10 minutes before relief of coronary occlusion in anesthetized swine; they also found improved coronary blood flow and fewer instances of no-reflow phenomenon.[31] Smalling and colleagues[32] demonstrated that support with IABP alone before relief of coronary occlusion could achieve infarct reductions of more than 40% in anesthetized dogs. Also in anesthetized dogs, Azevedo and colleagues[33] showed that LV unloading with IABP immediately before relief of coronary occlusion did not reduce infarct size (measured with cardiac MRI) but was associated with better regional wall motion and overall LV ejection fraction at 6 hours; these benefits were gone at 24 hours, however. Ventricular strain studies indicated IABP treatment did not reduce strain in transmural infarcts (about half the study regions in both treatment groups) but did reduce strain after 24 hours in regions with non-transmural

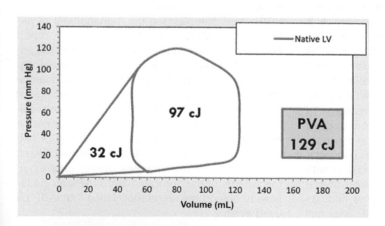

Fig. 4. Active (kinetic) and resting (potential) energy requirements for the LV. Under normal conditions, the pressure-volume area may account for about 100 cJ of total energy requirement, whereas the potential energy requirement is about one-third of this value. PVA, pressure-volume area. (*Courtesy of* CardiacAssist, Pittsburgh, PA; with permission.)

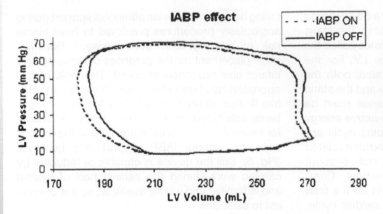

IABP effect

- - - - IABP ON
—— IABP OFF

Fig. 5. Pressure-volume loops in anesthetized sheep, with and without IABP support. (*From* Sauren LD, Accord RE, Hamzeh K, et al. Combined impella and intra-aortic balloon pump support to improve both ventricular unloading and coronary blood flow for myocardial recovery: an experimental study. Artif Organs 2007;31: 839–42; with permission.)

subendocardial infarction. The investigators concluded that IABP begun at the time of reperfusion accelerated recovery of contractility in reversibly injured regions; improved systolic contractility after 24 hours in segments with subendocardial infarction; improved global ventricular function early but not at 24 hours; and provided a small but significant improvement in systolic strain patterns over time. In sum, the animal studies of IABP support to improve ventricular salvage or performance during AMI yielded mixed results but sufficient signal of possible benefit to warrant consideration of human subject studies.

Few adequately sized human studies have been conducted to assess the impact of IABP on final infarct size. The best in this regard is the Counterpulsation Reduces Infarct Size Pre-PCI for AMI (CRISP-AMI) study by Patel and colleagues.[16] In this randomized clinical trial, 337 patients presenting with AMI without cardiogenic shock were assigned to receive PCI as usual (no IABP) or PCI following IABP placement. Infarct size measured at 3 to 5 days using cardiac MRI was the primary endpoint. About 80% of patients had adequate imaging studies. The results were surprising: mean infarct size was larger (42.1%, range 38.7%–45.6% of LV mass) with IABP than without it (37.5%, range, 34.3–40.8; the *P* value for this difference was .06), nearly significant in favor of no IABP. Similar calculations using median infarct sizes, and calculations using imputed values to account for patients who died before imaging, yielded similar results. Additionally, measures of LV dimensions and function were not improved with IABP. Despite this, mortality and the composite of death, shock, or heart failure over 6 months tended to be better for the patients treated with IABP, although these differences fell short of significance. Although the clinical outcome findings have caused some to argue that IABP may still

have a benefit, this study must be seen as evidence that routine use of IABP in patients with AMI without cardiogenic shock does not improve myocardial salvage, recovery, or function.

van't Hof and colleagues[34] conducted an earlier study that is also notable. This 3.5-year randomized controlled study involving 238 patients with AMI in The Netherlands found no benefit for IABP placement immediately after completion of primary angioplasty for AMI. Infarct size was estimated using the integral of lactate dehydrogenase release over 72 hours in about two-thirds of the patients and was not different between the two groups. Exactly the same percentage (26%) of patients in each group suffered an adverse clinical endpoint that made up the primary endpoint of the study. A high rate of crossover in both groups (25% in the IABP group, 31% in the control group) could have influenced the findings.

The clinical utility of IABP in the setting of cardiogenic shock has been assessed in many small studies, but the recent large ISAR SHOCK-II trial from Germany stands as perhaps the most definitive.[35] In this study, IABP placement had no beneficial effect on mortality or any secondary endpoints. The investigators concluded that IABP offers little value in the management of patients with AMI presenting with shock. A report on the experience in German clinical practice, assessed through a prospective national clinical registry of more than 55,000 patients with acute coronary syndromes, agreed with the findings of ISAR SHOCK-II.[36] Additionally, Sjauw and colleagues,[37] from The Netherlands, performed a meta-analysis of IABP value in the setting of AMI and concluded that the merit of their use seems so slim that the investigators openly challenged the authors of the European and American guidelines to defend the recommendation that IABP be used at all.

In summary, the published literature for the use of IABP to achieve reductions in infarct size or improved LV performance in human patients is discouraging. Although some patient subsets may find a benefit from the device, expectations should be limited. Despite some positive findings in some animal studies, there is little evidence that the use of IABP will reduce the size of myocardial injury meaningfully following AMI in humans (**Fig. 6**).

IMPELLA

The Impella device is a continuous axial flow pump placed retrograde across the aortic valve into the LV. Impella is presently available in the United States in 2 forms, the percutaneously implantable 2.5 system and the Impella 5.0, which requires surgical implantation. These devices are aptly named based on their maximum flow output in liters per minute. Because the focus of this review is the utility of devices available to the interventional cardiologist for quick placement during AMI, the discussion hereafter is limited to the Impella 2.5 device, except as noted. Impella is indicated for partial circulatory support for up to 6 hours.

Impella is placed in a manner similar to a pigtail catheter, which makes it appealing to invasive cardiologists. When compared with an IABP, the Impella takes less than 10 additional minutes to prime and place appropriately.[38] Impella is

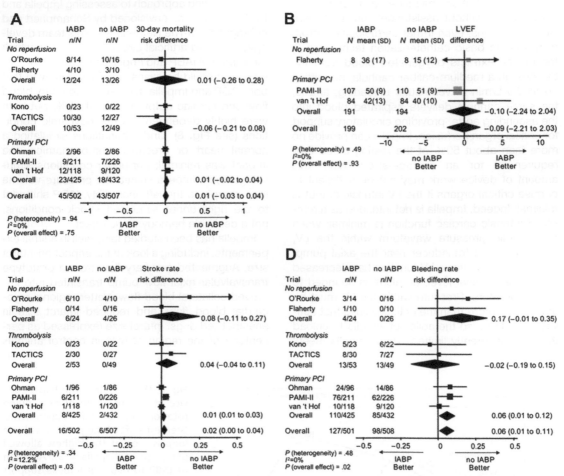

Fig. 6. Meta-analysis of impact of IABP placement before primary angioplasty in the setting of cardiogenic shock. (A) Impact on mortality at 30 days; (B) Impact on LV ejection fraction; (C) Impact on stroke; (D) Impact on bleeding complications. Colored squares with horizontal bars represent estimated treatment differences with 95% confidence intervals; diamond shapes represent the same information aggregated from the group of studies immediately above each diamond, compiled for meta-analysis. PAMI, Primary Angioplasty in Myocardial infarction; TACTICS, Treat Angina with aggrastat and determine Cost of Therapy with Invasive or Conservative Strategy. (*From* Sjauw KD, Engstrom AE, Vis MM, et al. A systematic review and meta-analysis of intra-aortic balloon pump therapy in ST-elevation myocardial infarction: should we change the guidelines? Eur Heart J 2009;30:459–68; with permission.)

contraindicated in patients with significant peripheral vascular disease, significant aortic disease (dissection or aneurysm), or tilting valve-type aortic valve replacement and should be used with caution in patients with aortic valve stenosis, ventricular thrombus, or ventricular septal defect. Impella has the unique feature of unloading the ventricle directly, resulting in lower LVEDP and LVEDV and reduced wall tension and myocardial oxygen consumption.[39] LV volume and pressure displacement are linearly correlated with the speed of rotation of the axial pump (**Fig. 7**). The continuous flow pump is not dependent on electrocardiographic or pressure triggers for activation. Impella approximates an ideal solution to the challenge of identifying a device to limit infarct size because (1) it can be placed by interventional cardiologists without assistance from perfusionists or surgeons, even if that cardiologist is proficient only in basic catheterization technique; (2) the device extracts oxygenated blood from the LV through a medium-caliber cannula, permitting up to 2.5 L/min of ventricular unloading; and (3) the same cannula delivers aspirated blood into the ascending aorta, providing circulatory support for critical organ perfusion. Impella can provide no more than about 50% of the resting blood flow requirement for an average-sized adult; this amount of device work may not be sufficient to perfuse critical organs if the LV intrinsic output is minimal. Indeed, Impella is not intended as a remedy if intrinsic cardiac function is minimal: when the systolic pressure waveform within the LV, measured by a transducer near the axial pump, discloses that intrinsic LV function has decreased less than a critical level, an alarm is sounded to notify operators. Pressure within the LV must be maintained more than the critical values that activate the alarm, so the ability of Impella to unload the LV is inherently limited. Thus, Impella meets some, but not all, of the chief requirements of an ideal solution for a percutaneous device to achieve infarct reduction.

Augmentation of coronary flow with Impella is thought to result from increased aortic perfusion pressure and decreased intramyocardial resistance from reduced LVEDV and microvasculature compression.[40] Coronary blood flow augmentation of 10% to 15% has been reported in animal studies.[41,42] In a comparative animal study, the ratio of stroke work to coronary blood flow was reduced by 69% with Impella and just 15% with IABP. The combination of Impella plus IABP lowered this ratio by 77%. The pulsatile effect of IABP may compliment the continuous perfusion provided by Impella.

A fascinating approach to assessing Impella and IABP support was envisioned by Schampaert and colleagues[42] in The Netherlands. This team developed a closed artificial circulation model in which the impact of IABP and Impella on modeled hemodynamics could be assessed. They observed that both IABP and Impella augmented coronary blood flow and cardiac output by about 10%, but both were highly dependent on hemodynamic conditions (see **Fig. 8**). Under conditions simulating a normal heart or preshock hemodynamics, the impact was minimal; but under conditions simulating shock, Impella shifted the pressure-volume loop sharply to the left. Incredibly, IABP shifted it to the right under simulated shock conditions, not a desirable hemodynamic effect.

Impella has been studied fairly well in animal experiments, including a look at the impact on infarct size. Augmented coronary flow from a prototype transvalvular axial flow pump translated into improved collateral blood flow, better regional myocardial blood flow, and reduced infarct size in anesthetized dogs. Infarct size (expressed as percentage of the region at risk) in control animals

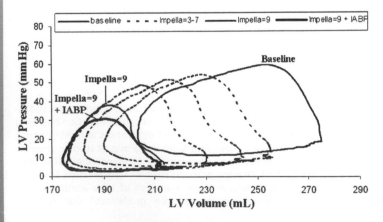

Fig. 7. LV unloading with Impella device at various speed of axial pump rotation in animal experiments. Greatest shift of the pressure-volume loop is seen at the highest allowed pump speed (Impella = 9). Addition of IABP to maximal Impella support effected small additional ventricular unloading. TLVA, transseptal LV assist. (*From* Schampaert S, van't Veer M, van de Vosse FN, et al. In vitro comparison of support capabilities of intra-aortic balloon pump and Impella 2.5 left percutaneous. Artif Organs 2011;35: 893–901; with permission.)

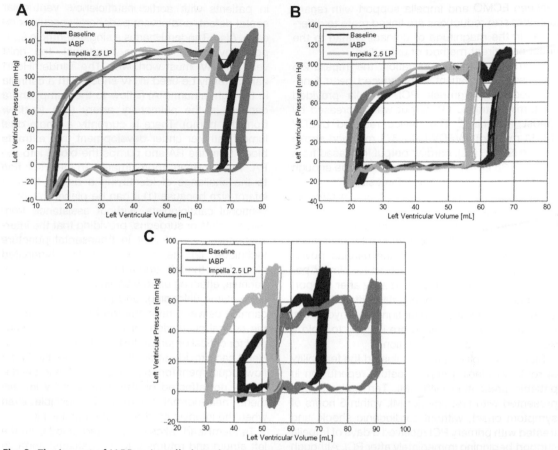

Fig. 8. The impact of IABP or Impella insertion on pressure-volume loops generated in a closed artificial circulation model, under various simulated conditions. (*A*) Simulated normal circulation. (*B*) Simulated preshock conditions. (*C*) Simulated cardiogenic shock conditions. (*From* Sauren LD, Accord RE, Hamzeh K, et al. Combined Impella and intra-aortic balloon pump support to improve both ventricular unloading and coronary blood flow for myocardial recovery: an experimental study. Artif Organs 2007;31:839–42; with permission.)

was 62.6%. With IABP support, this was reduced to 27% (*P* = .01). With the transvalvular axial flow pump, the infarct size was further reduced to 21.7% (*P* = .001). Although the transvalvular axial flow support proved superior to IABP, the magnitude of difference between the two was perhaps surprisingly small given the expected large difference in ventricular unloading possible between the two devices.

Infarct size was assessed in an ovine study conducted using Impella 5.0, but some experiments used this device at half power, which is roughly equivalent to maximal support from Impella 2.5.[32] Support was begun either before or after reperfusion. Infarct size (as a percentage of myocardium at risk) was 67% for control animals; this decreased to just 18% for animals supported before reperfusion with maximal Impella 5.0, to 42% with maximal Impella 5.0 support after reperfusion, and to 55% with Impella 5.0 at half power

after reperfusion. Myocardial oxygen consumption was significantly reduced with increasing LV support and was linearly related to final infarct size. Other experiments in dogs also showed that unloading the LV before, but not after, reperfusion reduced the extent of myocardial necrosis.[43] These experiments indicate that myocardial salvage depends on both the magnitude of unloading and the initiation of unloading before reperfusion.

A perceived benefit of Impella is that it unloads the LV directly. Some investigators have noted that ECMO is not effective in unloading the ventricle, which may be interpreted as failure of effectiveness of indirect LV unloading.[44,45] Interesting though, no differences in left ventricular end-systolic pressure (LVESP), systolic aortic pressure, or diastolic aortic pressure were observed between ECMO and Impella support in some animal studies.[44] It seems likely that any differences between ECMO and Impella support with regard to infarct size reductions are linked more to differences in the magnitude of unloading than to the direct or indirect method of unloading.

In an early human application, the Impella 2.5 was used in a patient with reduced heart function requiring high-risk PCI. Impella provided 2.4 L/min; intrinsic LV output was decreased by almost 1 L/min.[46] The device reduced LVEDP (18–11 mm Hg), LVEDV (345–321 mL), and stroke volume (94–76 mL); cardiac output increased from 5.95 to 7.38 L/min. This increase might be enough to effect a reduction in final infarct size.

The impact of Impella support begun after reperfusion was studied in a small number of patients who presented with cardiogenic shock complicating AMI.[38] The important observation for this discussion was that the cardiac power index was significantly better than for similar patients treated with IABP immediately after support was begun, but by 2 hours this difference was gone. Short-duration reductions in myocardial strain and oxygen demand are unlikely to yield a meaningful infarct size reduction.

Sjauw and colleagues[47] evaluated the feasibility of routinely placing Impella before reperfusion in patients presenting with AMI. Ten patients who presented with first anterior MI, within 6 hours of symptom onset, without cardiogenic shock, and treated with primary PCI received 3 days of Impella support beginning immediately after PCI. Although the cardiac output and pulmonary capillary wedge pressure improved with Impella compared with concurrent patients treated with IABP, differences were not significant. Relative improvement in LV ejection fraction at 3 days and 4 months was greater for Impella patients than IABP patients, although Impella patients had much worse LVEF at baseline. Additional and adequately powered studies are required to demonstrate the effect of Impella usage on infarct size in ST-segment elevation MI (STEMI). The arrival of Impella CP, capable of delivering >3.7 L/min, is likely to perform better than the 2.5 version and does not require a cut down like the 5.0 Impella device.

TANDEMHEART

TandemHeart is a percutaneous LV support device approved for short-term use (6 hours). A transseptal technique is used to deploy the cannula in the left atrium.[48] A maximum pumping rate of 5 L/min is possible, depending on the size of cannulae used and the loading conditions. TandemHeart is indicated clinically for short-term stabilization of patients following cardiogenic shock complicating AMI. The device is contraindicated in patients with aortic insufficiency, ventricular septal defect, and severe peripheral vascular disease. Also, TandemHeart is a single-ventricle support device; for it to be functional, the right ventricle (RV) must work well. The TandemHeart can currently be used in RV shock with a cannula in the right atrium (RA) (inflow to the pump) and a cannula in the pulmonary artery (PA) (outflow from the pump). There is currently a single dual lumen catheter under development that extracts blood from the RA and pumps the blood into the PA. TandemHeart approximates an ideal solution to the challenge of identifying a device to limit infarct size because (1) it can be placed by interventional cardiologists, without assistance from perfusionists or surgeons, providing that the interventionalist is proficient in transseptal puncture technique; (2) the device extracts oxygenated blood from the left atrium through a large-caliber cannula, effecting up to 5 L/min of indirect ventricular volume unloading; and (3) the arterial return cannula delivers the extracted blood volume into the central circulation, providing circulatory support for critical organ perfusion. Because TandemHeart can provide about 80% of the resting blood flow requirement for an average adult, and the device is not affected by the degree of LV impairment, near-normal perfusion is possible even when the intrinsic cardiac contribution is nil.

TandemHeart takes oxygenated blood from the left atrium and returns it to the patients' aorta, in essence, a left atrium-to-descending aorta LV bypass. Unlike Impella, TandemHeart relieves the LV indirectly by depleting the left atrial blood volume available to enter the LV during diastole. The theoretical limit of the volume of blood that can be drained indirectly from the LV is nearly twice the theoretical limit of the volume of blood that the Impella 2.5 can drain directly from the LV; although there are no direct comparative studies to date, the greater flow achieved with the TandemHeart suggests that it might have a greater effect than the Impella 2.5 on the LV pressure-volume relationship because of greater unloading. The Impella 5.0 (not a percutaneous device) or the CP Impella (4.0 L/min) might be expected to have similar unloading compared with the TandemHeart. These types of studies are likely to be forthcoming and will help elucidate these issues.

The theoretical effect of TandemHeart support on the LV pressure-volume relationship is shown in **Fig. 9**. Most of the work of generating cardiac output is relieved with TandemHeart, and even passive energy requirements are reduced slightly. Compared with normal conditions, TandemHeart is capable of lowering total LV energy

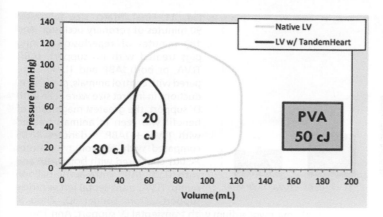

Fig. 9. Illustration of LV pressure-volume relationship with Tandem-Heart device support. As the ventricle is unloaded, systolic and diastolic pressure within the ventricle decreases, and the diminished pressure-volume loop shifts to the left. Passive (potential) energy requirement is diminished slightly. Overall, a reduction of more than 60% of LV energy requirement is possible. (*Courtesy of* CardiacAssist, Pittsburgh, PA; with permission.)

requirements from about 130 cJ to around 50 cJ, that is, a reduction of more than 60%. If this theoretical hemodynamic circumstance is a close approximation to actual conditions, then unloading of the LV to a range shown to provide meaningful infarct size reductions is possible.

As mentioned earlier, some have questioned the value of indirect LV unloading in view of the poor results of LV unloading with ECMO. The impact on the pressure-volume loop is greater for TandemHeart than with ECMO, perhaps because ECMO must draw from the highly compliant vena cavae (limiting the maximal blood draw rate) and pass the blood through a membrane oxygenator (increasing flow resistance). As a result, the pressure-volume loop is shifted down and to the left when TandemHeart support replaces ECMO support in animal studies (see **Fig. 10**).

Left atrial to femoral artery bypass was shown to reduce myocardial infarct size and improve survival following coronary artery occlusion in an experimental animal model as early as 1983.[49] Fonger and colleagues[27] conducted an important, and relevant, subsequent animal study.[27] In this study, 32 pigs undergoing conditions intended to simulate cardiopulmonary bypass for cardiac surgery were assigned to one of 4 groups: (1) no support (control); (2) support with an IABP; (3) support with transseptal LV assist (TLVA) using a cannula and pumping system similar to the TandemHeart system; and (4) support with both IABP and TLVA. Support was provided for 90 minutes of coronary occlusion and continued for 180 minutes after reperfusion. Support lowered LVEDP and was associated with a reduction in final infarct size, although the impact of IABP was less than with TLVA (**Fig. 11**). Interestingly, the combination of IABP and TLVA provided the greatest benefit: the area of infarct was reduced to just 6.7% ± 1.9% of the area at risk (see **Fig. 11**). Regional wall motion, however, was not improved with any support.

Navin Kapur, at Tufts University, completed recent important animal work. Using a pig model of MI, Kapur assessed LV pressure-volume loops at baseline, during coronary occlusion, and after reperfusion (**Fig. 12**). As expected, coronary occlusion caused a shift of the pressure-volume loop to the right, an increase in diastolic pressures, and a decrease in the systolic peak pressures. Reperfusion without LV support caused further

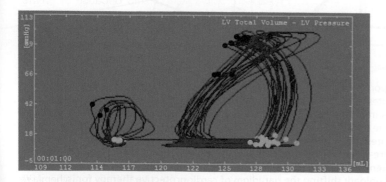

Fig. 10. Pressure-volume loops from animal experiment assessing impact of ECMO and TandemHeart. Pressure-volume loop to the right is taken under conditions of ECMO support. The loop to the left is from the same animal supported with TandemHeart left atrium to aorta (LA-Ao) bypass. *Red lines* represent pressure-volume measurements over multiple cardiac cycles. *Blue dots* represent end-systolic values. *Green dots* represent end-diastolic values. (*Courtesy of* CardiacAssist, Pittsburgh, PA; with permission.)

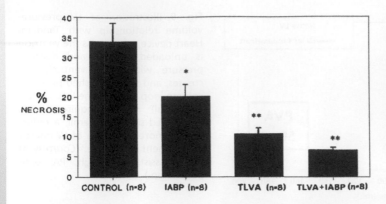

Fig. 11. Final infarct size following 90 minutes of coronary occlusion and 180 minutes of reperfusion among pigs treated with no support, IABP, TLVA, or both IABP and TLVA. Compared with control animals, marked reductions in infarct size were seen with LV support, the greatest magnitude of benefit was seen in animals treated with TLVA + IABP. * denotes P<.05 compared with control. ** denotes P<.001 compared with both IABP and with TLVA. IABP, intra-aortic balloon pump; TLVA, trans-septal left ventricle support. (*From* Fonger JD, Zhou Y, Matsuura H, et al. Enhanced preservation of acutely ischemic myocardium with transseptal LV support. Ann Thorac Surg 1994;57:570–5; with permission.)

worsening of this pattern, with significant additional LV dilatation and pump impairment. In contrast, reperfusion with TandemHeart support caused the pressure-volume loop to collapse down and to the left as LV volume and pressure were sharply reduced. LV stroke work was reduced to about 15% of the baseline with TandemHeart support, greatly reducing regional and circumferential myocardial strain. In addition, activation of the RISK pathway prosurvival kinases were assessed. Although experimental AMI without support did not activate these enzymes, AMI with LV unloading did (**Fig. 13**). Finally, histologic and biochemical analyses confirmed large reductions in the area of injury among those animals receiving LV unloading with reperfusion; the area of myocardial injury was linearly related to the stroke work required of intrinsic LV function (**Fig. 14**).

No studies have been conducted in human patients to assess if LV unloading during AMI with TandemHeart can reduce infarct size. To determine if this is possible, a randomized clinical trial has been launched: the TandemHeart to Reduce Infarct Size trial (see **Fig. 10**). Initially envisioned as a European study, this trial has received approval from Food and Drug Administration to move ahead in the United States. The study will begin with a feasibility phase; during this phase, 50 patients presenting to one of 5 participating hospitals within 12 hours of the onset of chest pain will undergo primary PCI after the Tandem-Heart device has been placed and the LV is unloaded. This feasibility phase is needed to determine if operators can place the device in such patients adequately and to understand the additional time required for device placement in this setting. Even if TandemHeart unloading

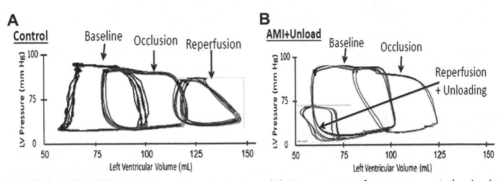

Fig. 12. Pressure-volume loops from porcine experiments. (*A*) Measurements from unsupported animals under baseline conditions following 60 minutes of coronary occlusion and after reperfusion. Unsupported reperfusion is associated with deleterious changes in LV pressure-volume loops. (*B*) Measurements from animals supported with TandemHeart device under baseline conditions following 60 minutes of coronary occlusion and after reperfusion. TandemHeart support shifts the pressure-volume loop sharply down and to the left, a very favorable hemodynamic effect. *Lines* represent pressure volume measurements over multiple cardiac cycles. *Blue dots* represent end-systolic values. *Green dots* represent end-diastolic values. (*Data from* Kapur NK, Paruchuri V, Mackey EE, et al. From door to balloon to door to unload: shifting the paradigm of cardioprotective therapy for ischemia reperfusion injury in acute myocardial infarction [abstract]. Circulation 2012;126:A16199.)

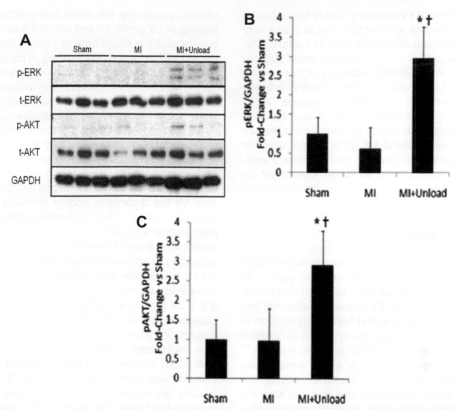

Fig. 13. Rapid induction of salvage pathway kinases with LV unloading. (*A*) Gel electrophoresis demonstrating induction of p-ERK and p-AKT bands (salvage pathway kinases) under conditions of AMI with ventricular unloading with TandemHeart, but not under sham conditions or AMI without unloading. (*B*) Compared with sham (control) or AMI without unloading, AMI with unloading results in approximately 3-fold increase in levels of p-ERK and p-AKT (normalized for control protein concentrations). GAPDH, glyceraldehyde-3 phosphate dehydrogenase; p-AKT, protein kinase B; p-ERK, phosphorylated extracellular signal-regulated kinase. (*Data from* Kapur NK, Paruchuri V, Mackey EE, et al. From door to balloon to door to unload: shifting the paradigm of cardioprotective therapy for ischemia reperfusion injury in acute myocardial infarction [abstract]. Circulation 2012;126:A16199.)

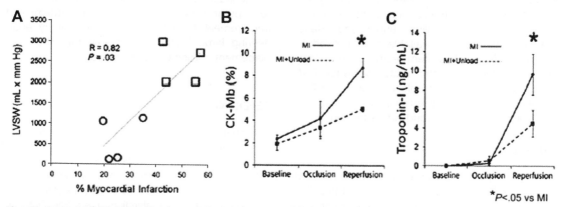

Fig. 14. Impact of LV unloading in experimental AMI model. (*A*) Relationship between LV stroke work and final infarct size. Circles indicate with LV unloading; squares indicate control animals. (*B*) Impact of LV unloading on CK-Mb release. (*C*) Impact of LV unloading on troponin release. CK-Mb, combined serum concentration of creatine kinase isozymes M and B. (*Data from* Kapur NK, Paruchuri V, Mackey EE, et al. From door to balloon to door to unload: shifting the paradigm of cardioprotective therapy for ischemia reperfusion injury in acute myocardial infarction [abstract]. Circulation 2012;126:A16199.)

greatly enhanced LV recovery, a very long delay to relief of coronary obstruction could mask any benefit. Assuming this phase passes successfully, the architects of the trial intend to enroll 200 patients assigned randomly to primary PCI or primary PCI plus TandemHeart. The primary efficacy endpoint will be myocardial salvage index measured by cardiac MRI within 5 days of treatment. A composite safety endpoint will measure rates of death, repeat MI, stroke, and vascular complications at 30 days, 6 months, and 1 year. This study is expected to begin enrollment by summer 2013 and should be completed within 36 months.

FUTURE DEVICES

At least one other device is under development for LV support, although the therapeutic goal is to improve stability rather than reduce infarct size. Thoratec Corporation (Pleasanton, California) has recently announced the first human application of their Percutaneous Heart Pump (PHP) to support 3 patients during high-risk PCI in South America.[50] The PHP is inserted through a 12F sheath: one French size smaller than the sheath required for Impella and 3 French sizes smaller than the smallest TandemHeart arterial cannula. PHP has an elastomeric, collapsible impeller and cannula that, unlike Impella, is driven by an external motor attached to a thin drive shaft. The expandable components are positioned across the aortic valve and expanded to a 24F diameter. With the much larger dimensions, PHP can displace as much as 5 L/min at low rotational speeds, eliminating concerns over significant hemolysis. This tool could potentially address concerns about Impella (insufficient LV unloading, limited by hemolysis and catheter diameter) and about TandemHeart (transseptal puncture requirement, very large indwelling venous and arterial cannulae). No data are available on infarct reduction with PHP, but the system seems to have promise. Also, the new and more powerful FDA approved Impella CP is able to provide >3.7 L/min of flow. Proper designed clinical trials are however mandatory before worldwide adoption.

SUMMARY

Improving myocyte salvage during AMI has proved elusive; the keys to success seem to be the ability to lower oxygen demand of ischemic myocardium and also activate salvage enzyme pathways to take advantage of endogenous cardioprotective mechanisms. Pharmacologic approaches have been largely unsuccessful. Early work by surgeons interested in salvaging myocardium injured during cardiac operations identified that mechanical unloading of LV pressure and volume improved outcomes, and the magnitude of benefit was directly related to the degree of unloading. A percutaneous LV assist device could improve myocyte salvage during AMI therapy if it was able to reduce myocardial oxygen demand, wall tension, and LV stroke work substantially. An ideal device should be readily manageable by a catheterization laboratory team, reduce LV stroke work by more than 50%, and sustain adequate systemic perfusion to maintain organ viability even when intrinsic cardiac function is minimal, in addition to reducing infarct size. Of the 3 devices widely available in North America, only the IABP has been best tested in human studies to determine its ability to reduce final infarct size; it was found to provide insufficient LV unloading to achieve this goal. Impella 2.5 unloads the LV to a greater extent than the IABP, and TandemHeart unloads the LV more than the Impella 2.5. Both Impella and TandemHeart are in the early phases of human patient clinical studies aimed at determining if they can interfere with lethal reperfusion injury and programed cell death following AMI. Both devices are being assessed for feasibility of use in the setting of AMI; if feasibility studies are successful, pivotal efficacy trials are expected to follow. The results of the randomized clinical trials of the Impella devices and the TandemHeart in AMI are eagerly awaited. The technical challenge of placing the more demanding TandemHeart quickly in patients with AMI could limit acceptance by physicians, especially those who are not facile with transseptal puncture. Animal data indicate that beginning LV support before reperfusion provides the greatest opportunity for benefit. Future devices will focus on overcoming the limitations of Impella (hemolysis with faster axial pump rotational speeds) and TandemHeart (requirement for transseptal puncture) by engineering larger catheters suitable for retrograde placement across the aortic valve.

REFERENCES

1. Forrester JS, Wyatt HL, Da Luz PL, et al. Functional significance of regional ischemic contraction abnormalities. Circulation 1976;54:64–70.
2. Oh JK, Ding ZP, Gersh BJ, et al. Restrictive LV diastolic filling identifies patients with heart failure after acute myocardial infarction. J Am Soc Echocardiogr 1992;5(5):497–503.
3. Moller JE, Whalley GA, Dini FL, et al. Independent prognostic importance of a restrictive LV filling pattern after myocardial infarction: an individual patient meta-analysis: meta analysis research

group in echocardiography acute myocardial infarction. Circulation 2008;117:2591–8.

4. Hillis GS, Moller JE, Pellikka PA, et al. Noninvasive estimation of left ventricular filling pressure by E/e' is a powerful predictor of survival after acute myocardial infarction. J Am Coll Cardiol 2004;43: 360–7.

5. Møller JE, Egstrup K, Køber L, et al. Prognostic importance of systolic and diastolic function after acute myocardial infarction. Am Heart J 2003; 145:147–53.

6. Ersboll M, Andersen MJ, Valeur N, et al. The prognostic value of left atrial peak pressure reservoir strain in acute myocardial infarction is dependent on left ventricular longitudinal function and left atrial size. Circ Cardiovasc Imaging 2013;6:26–33.

7. Klabunde RE. Cardiovascular physiology concepts. 2nd edition. Philadelphia: Lippincott Williams and Wilkins; 2011.

8. Ardehali A, Ports TA. Myocardial oxygen supply and demand. Chest 1990;98(3):699–705.

9. Berne RM. The role of adenosine in the regulation of coronary blood flow. Circ Res 1980;47:807–13.

10. Mosher P, Ross PJ Jr, McFate PA, et al. Control of coronary blood flow by an autoregulatory mechanism. Circ Res 1964;14:250–9.

11. Downey JM, Kirk ES. Distribution of the coronary blood flow across the canine heart wall during systole. Circ Res 1974;34:251–7.

12. Lewis FB, Coffmann JD, Gregg DE. Effect of heart rate and intracoronary isoproterenol, levarterenol, and epinephrine on coronary flow and resistance. Circ Res 1961;9:89–95.

13. Neil WA, Oxendine J, Phelps N, et al. Subendocardial ischemia provoked by tachycardia in conscious dogs with coronary stenosis. Am J Cardiol 1975;35: 30–6.

14. Yellon DM, Hausenloy DJ. Myocardial reperfusion injury. N Engl J Med 2007;357:1121–35.

15. Piot C, Croisille P, Staat P. Effect of cyclosporine on reperfusion injury in acute myocardial infarction. N Engl J Med 2008;359:473–81.

16. Patel MR, Smalling RW, Thiele H, et al. Intra-aortic balloon counterpulsation and infarct size in patients with acute anterior myocardial infarction without shock: the CRISP AMI randomized trial. JAMA 2011;306(12):1329–37.

17. Kristen AV, Ackermann K, Buss S, et al. Inhibition of apoptosis by the intrinsic but not the extrinsic apoptotic pathway in myocardial ischemia-reperfusion. Cardiovasc Pathol 2013. http://dx.doi.org/10.1016/j.carpath.2013.01.004. pii:S1054–8807(13)00007-0.

18. Wajant H. The Fas signaling pathway: more than a paradigm. Science 2002;296(31):1653–6.

19. Llu F, Bardhan K, Yang D, et al. NF-κB directly regulates Fas transcription to modulate Fas-mediated apoptosis and tumor suppression. J Biol Chem 2012;287:25530–40.

20. Hausenloy DJ, Yellon DM. New directions for protecting the heart against ischaemia/reperfusion injury: targeting the reperfusion injury salvage kinase (RISK) pathway. Cardiovasc Res 2004;61:448–60.

21. Davidson SM, Hausenloy D, Duchen MR, et al. Singalling via the reperfusion injury signaling kinase (RISK) pathway links closure of the mitochondrial permeability transition pore to cardioprotection. Int J Biochem Cell Biol 2006;38:414–9.

22. Hausenloy DJ, Yellon DM. The mitochondrial permeability transition pore: its fundamental role in mediating cell death during ischaemia and reperfusion. J Mol Cell Cardiol 2003;35:339–41.

23. du Toit EF, Genis A, Opie LH, et al. A role for the RISK pathway and KATP channels in pre- and post-conditioning induced by levosimendan in the isolated guinea pig heart. Br J Pharmacol 2008; 154:41–50.

24. Ross AM, Gibbons RJ, Stone GW, et al. A randomized double-blinded, placebo-controlled multicenter trial of adenosine as an adjunct to reperfusion in the treatment of acute myocardial infarction (AMISTAD-II). J Am Coll Cardiol 2005; 45(11):1775–80.

25. Kloner RA, Forman MB, Gibbons RJ, et al. Impact of time to therapy and reperfusion modality on the efficacy of adenosine in acute myocardial infarction: the AMISTAD-2 trial. Eur Heart J 2006; 27(20):2400–5.

26. Cohen MV, Downey JM. Adenosine: trigger and mediator of cardioprotection. Basic Res Cardiol 2008;103:203–15.

27. Fonger JD, Zhou Y, Matsuura H, et al. Enhanced preservation of acutely ischemic myocardium with transseptal LV support. Ann Thorac Surg 1994;57: 570–5.

28. Khalafbeigui F, Suga H, Sagawa K. Left ventricular systolic pressure-volume area correlates with oxygen consumption. Am J Physiol 1979;237(5): H566–9.

29. Brodie BR, Stuckey TD, Hansen C, et al. Intra-aortic balloon counterpulsation before primary percutaneous angioplasty reduces catheterization laboratory events in high-risk patients with acute myocardial infarction. Am J Cardiol 1999;84:18–23.

30. Cyrus T, Mathews SJ, Lasala JM. Use of mechanical assist during high-risk PCI and STEMI with cardiogenic shock. Catheter Cardiovasc Interv 2010;75(Suppl 1):S1–6.

31. Pierrakos CN, Bonios MJ, Drakos SG, et al. Mechanical assistance by intra-aortic balloon pump counterpulsation during reperfusion increases coronary blood flow and mitigates the no-reflow phenomenon: an experimental study. Artif Organs 2011;35:867–74.

32. Smalling RW, Cassidy DB, Barrett R, et al. Improved regional myocardial blood flow, left ventricular unloading, and infarct salvage using an axial-flow, transvalvular left ventricular assist device. A comparison with intra-aortic balloon counterpulsation and reperfusion alone in a canine infarction model. Circulation 1992;85(3):1152–9.

33. Azevedo CF, Amado LC, Kraitchman DL, et al. The effect of intra-aortic balloon counterpulsation on left ventricular functional recovery early after acute myocardial infarction: a randomized experimental magnetic resonance imaging study. Eur Heart J 2005;26:1235–41.

34. van 't Hof AW, Liem AL, de Boer MJ, et al. A randomized comparison of intra-aortic balloon pumping after primary coronary angioplasty in high risk patients with acute myocardial infarction. Eur Heart J 1999;20(9):659–65.

35. Thiele H, Zeymer U, Neumann FJ, et al. Intraaortic balloon support for myocardial infarction with cardiogenic shock. N Engl J Med 2012;367:1287–96.

36. Zeyman U, Hochadel M, Hauptmann KE, et al. Intra-aortic balloon pump in patients with acute myocardial infarction complicated by cardiogenic shock: results of the ALKK-PCI registry. Clin Res Cardiol 2013;103:223–7.

37. Sjauw KD, Engstrom AE, Vis MM, et al. A systematic review and meta-analysis of intra-aortic balloon pump therapy in ST-elevation myocardial infarction: should we change the guidelines? Eur Heart J 2009;30:459–68.

38. Seyfarth M, Sibbing D, Bauer I, et al. A randomized clinical trial to evaluate the safety and efficacy of a percutaneous left ventricular assist device versus intra-aortic balloon pumping for treatment of cardiogenic shock caused by myocardial infarction. J Am Coll Cardiol 2008;52:1584–8.

39. Morley D, Litwak K, Ferber P, et al. Hemodynamic effects of partial ventricular support in chronic heart failure: results of simulation validated with in vivo data. J Thorac Cardiovasc Surg 2007;133:21–8.

40. Remmelink M, Sjauw KD, Yong ZY, et al. Coronary microcirculatory dysfunction is associated with left ventricular dysfunction during follow-up after STEMI. Neth Heart J 2013;21(5):238–44.

41. Sauren LD, Accord RE, Hamzeh K, et al. Combined Impella and intra-aortic balloon pump support to improve both ventricular unloading and coronary blood flow for myocardial recovery: an experimental study. Artif Organs 2007;31:839–42.

42. Schampaert S, van't Veer M, van de Vosse FN, et al. In vitro comparison of support capabilities of intra-aortic balloon pump and Impella 2.5 left percutaneous. Artif Organs 2011;35:893–901.

43. Achour H, Boccalandro F, Felli P, et al. Mechanical left ventricular unloading prior to reperfusion reduces infarct size in a canine infarction model. Catheter Cardiovasc Interv 2005;64(2):182–92.

44. Kawashima D, Gojo S, Nishimura T, et al. Left ventricular mechanical support with Impella provides more ventricular unloading in heart failure than extracorporeal membrane oxygenation. ASAIO J 2011;57(3):169–76.

45. Koeckert MS, Jorde UP, Naka Y, et al. 2.5 for LV unloading during venoarterial extracorporeal membrane oxygenation support. J Cardiovasc Surg 2011;26:666–8.

46. Valgimigli M, Steendijk P, Sianos G, et al. Left ventricular unloading and concomitant total cardiac output increase by the use of percutaneous Impella Recover LP 2.5 assist device during high risk coronary intervention. Catheter Cardiovasc Interv 2005; 65:263–7.

47. Sjauw KD, Remmelink M, Baan J Jr, et al. Left ventricular unloading in acute ST-segment elevation myocardial infarction patients is safe and feasible and provides acute and sustained left ventricular recovery. J Am Coll Cardiol 2008; 51(10):1044–6.

48. Vranckx P, Foley DP, de Feijter PJ, et al. Clinical introduction of the Tandem Heart, a percutaneous left ventricular assist device, for circulatory support during high-risk percutaneous coronary intervention. Int J Cardiovasc Intervent 2003;5:35–9.

49. Catinella P, Cunningham JN, Glassman E, et al. Left atrium to femoral bypass: effectiveness in reduction of acute experimental myocardial infarction. J Thorac Cardiovasc Surg 1983;86:887–96.

50. Available at: http://phx.corporate-ir.net/phoenix.zhtml?c=95989&p=irol-news&nyo=0.

Future Directions for Percutaneous Mechanical Circulatory Support Devices

Tim Lockie, MBChB, PhD[a],
Simon Redwood, MD, FRCP, FACC, FSCAI[b],*

KEYWORDS

- Percutaneous mechanical support • Cardiogenic shock • Novel
- Integrated circulatory support network • Future • Novel device technology

KEY POINTS

- The development of novel percutaneous mechanical circulatory support devices offers additional therapeutic options for patients in cardiogenic shock.
- Hand in hand with innovations in device technology must also come development of integrated circulatory support networks focusing on rapid assessment of patients, multidisciplinary discussion, and timely therapeutic intervention.
- Miniaturization of technology means increasingly powerful devices are available with smaller shaft size, minimizing entry site complications and facilitating insertion. Options for percutaneous right ventricular support are also in development, as well as mobile ECMO devices that offer the possibility of full life support and inter-hospital transfer.

INTRODUCTION

Despite prompt revascularization, pharmacologic treatment, and the use of the intra-aortic balloon pump (IABP) therapy, the rate of mortality in cardiogenic shock patients remains high.[1] A recent editorial in the *New England Journal of Medicine* discussing the findings of the IABP-SHOCK II trial[2] concluded that despite the negative findings of this trial that compared the outcome of 600 patients with IABP with standard therapy in cardiogenic shock complicating ST segment elevation myocardial infarction (STEMI), that "we must move forward with the understanding that a cardiovascular condition with 40% mortality at 30 days remains unacceptable."[3] The experience in novel mechanical circulatory support (MCS) therapy, however, is

expanding rapidly. Currently available percutaneous mechanical circulatory support (pMCS) devices are promising and safety and feasibility studies are encouraging in patients with cardiogenic shock.[4] As device design continues to improve with greater longevity, reduced size, and reduction in insertion point complications, the range of patients that may be suitable for these devices and the indications for their use may be expected to continue to increase. In advanced heart failure patients, pMCS devices may select patients who would benefit from long-term, durable MCS therapy either as a bridge-to-transplant[5] or in patients not suitable for transplant, as destination therapy in its own right.[6] In patients with cardiogenic shock, pMCS can provide immediate

Funding Sources: T. Lockie, Guys & St Thomas' NHS Trust, London, UK. S. Redwood, KCL, London.
Conflicts of Interest: None.
^a Cardiothoracic Centre, St Thomas' Hospital, Guys & St Thomas' NHS Trust, Westminster Bridge Road, London SE1 7EH, UK; ^b King's College London British Heart Foundation Centre of Excellence, The Rayne Institute, St Thomas' Hospital Campus, London, UK
* Corresponding author. Cardiothoracic Centre, St Thomas' Hospital, 6th Floor East Wing, London SE1 7EH, UK.
E-mail address: Simon.Redwood@gstt.nhs.uk

Intervent Cardiol Clin 2 (2013) 485–494
http://dx.doi.org/10.1016/j.iccl.2013.03.004
2211-7458/13/$ – see front matter © 2013 Published by Elsevier Inc.

because it was devised in an era that preceded the use of contemporary heart failure therapy such as aldosterone antagonists, defibrillators, and cardiac resynchronization therapy. The Seattle Heart Failure Model[12] is predictive of mortality in heart failure and may be used to identify at-risk patients and may be more representative of the current treated heart failure population. It is hoped that the use of such risk stratification models can be used in future clinical trials involving MCS to provide further validation of their use, as such data are currently lacking.[13,14] In hospitalized patients the Acute Decompensated Heart Failure National Registry[15] provides a predictive model for heart failure patients at admission based on 3 readily available variables including systolic blood pressure <115 mm Hg, blood urea nitrogen ≥43 mg/dL, and serum creatinine ≥2.75 mg/dL. In this analysis, the in-hospital mortality varies from 2.1% for the low-risk group to 21.9% in the high-risk group. The Interagency Registry for Mechanically Assisted Circulatory Support (INTERMACS) is a US registry accumulating data on patients following US Food and Drug Administration (FDA)–approved MCS device implantation. Within INTERMACS, patients are classified by their signs and symptoms into different clinical profiles.[16] This classification differentiates patients with New York Heart Association (NYHA) class III to IV symptoms and provides a more detailed description of disease severity. The prognostic implications of the INTERMACS profiles provide guidance for the optimal timing of implantation and the associated risks based on clinical presentation and are being investigated in several clinical trials.[17–19] Several other databases also provide descriptions of risk factors for mortality after MCS implantation. These databases include the Columbia University/Cleveland Clinic risk factor selection,[20] and the Muenster risk score.[21] The Lietz-Miller score is a tool to assess longer-term mortality after implantation of durable MCS based on data from 280 patients who underwent implantation of the pulsatile HeartMate XVE left ventricular assist device.[22] This risk model has not yet been validated with continuous-flow devices.

Ultimately the decision to implant MCS in a patient must be based on a comprehensive multidisciplinary assessment of the patient's clinical condition and associated co-morbidities; their social situation at home; quality of life; and, importantly, their and their family's wishes and expectations. All of this should be interpreted in the context of the experience and availability of resources within the treating center. There is a need for more prospective models to the guide the timing of and risk associated with implantation to provide a more robust and objective approach to patient selection for MCS.

Assessing Outcomes of MCS Therapy

The ability to maintain hemodynamic stability remains a primary objective of MCS in cardiogenic shock. In particular, this means reaching and maintaining a physiologically appropriate mean arterial pressure, cardiac output, and pulmonary venous pressure for the given clinical state while ensuring adequate organ perfusion at the tissue level. Characterizing targets for each of these parameters can be challenging, resulting in patients receiving either insufficient or excessive support, with consequent poor outcome.[23] The prognostic ability of a novel hemodynamic parameter, cardiac power output (CPO) measured in watts, has been examined.[24] This parameter is defined as the mean arterial pressure multiplied by the cardiac output and divided by 451. It accounts for the growing belief that cardiac output alone is not sufficient for end-organ perfusion; adequate mean arterial pressure also seems to be required. Several studies have examined the prognostic power of this novel hemodynamic parameter. CPO was able to predict mortality in various cardiac conditions, including cardiogenic shock secondary to acute myocardial infarction, both ischemic and nonischemic cardiomyopathy, and fulminant[25] myocarditis.[20,21] In patients without shock, CPO was able to predict clinical deterioration and death in patients admitted with decompensated heart failure.[26] In these same studies, neither cardiac output alone nor other more traditional parameters such as mean arterial pressure or pulmonary venous pressure were independently associated with mortality.

Importantly, certain minimum CPO cutoff points have now emerged as potential predictors of outcome, whereby if CPO decreases to below these levels, then poor outcome can be expected.[24] Although these values still need to be validated in a prospective fashion, from a hemodynamic point of view, an MCS device should be set up to maintain CPO levels above these cutoffs to maintain hemodynamic stability and improve tissue perfusion, and hence, survival. The ideal device would be selected to achieve these targets without additional vasopressor or inotropic therapy and thereby avoid the adverse outcome associated with these agents.[23,27]

FUTURE DEVICE DEVELOPMENT FOR PERCUTANEOUS MCS

Once it has been decided that the patient is a candidate for pMCS, then the appropriate device needs to be selected. Currently the available devices include the IABP, the Impella LP 2.5 and LP 5 (Abiomed, Inc, Danvers, MA, USA), and the TandemHeart (CardiacAssist, Inc, Pittsburgh, PA, USA). External counterpulsation devices have been used since the 1970s, mostly for intractable angina but also in cardiogenic shock.[28] Percutaneous extracorporeal membrane oxygenation (ECMO) systems can also be used for cardiopulmonary support as an acute bridge to therapy or myocardial recovery in cardiogenic shock.[29] Some further devices currently in development are discussed later.

Left Ventricular Support Devices

The HeartMate PHP (Percutaneous Heart Pump; Thoratec, Pleasanton, CA, USA) device is an axial flow pump currently under development. It is inserted through an 11-F introducer sheath that is expandable to 21 F, with an elastomeric, collapsible impeller and cannula that is driven by an external motor via a flexible drive shaft. In a laboratory setting, the device has generated greater than 4.5 L per minute of flow against normal physiologic pressures.

The Impella cVAD (Abiomed, Danvers, MA) has recently received CE Marking approval for use in the European Union and is also available in Canada. It is a truly percutaneous device without the need for surgical intervention that can deliver blood flow up to 4 L/min and can be left in situ for up to 5 days (**Fig. 1**).

The Reitan Catheter Pump (CardioBridge) consists of a catheter-mounted pump-head with a foldable propeller and surrounding cage (**Fig. 2**). It is positioned in the descending aorta where the pump creates a pressure gradient, reducing afterload and enhancing organ perfusion. The first small series of the use of this device have been published[30] but further clinical evaluation is awaited.

In addition, the iVAC 3L device (PulseCath BV, Amsterdam, the Netherlands) is a 17-F or 21-F catheter with an integrated 2-way valve system that pulls blood from the left ventricle (LV) and delivers it to the ascending aorta and is driven by a standard IABP console (**Fig. 3**). It is capable of generating pulsatile flow of 2 to 3 L/min. It has been used successfully in individual patients for cardiopulmonary bypass during coronary artery bypass grafting.[31]

Currently available percutaneous devices are only able to provide short-duration MCS. Development of percutaneous durable devices is also underway, such as the SYNERGY Micro-pump (CircuLite, Inc, Saddle Brook, NJ, USA), that would be positioned in a subcutaneous pocket over the

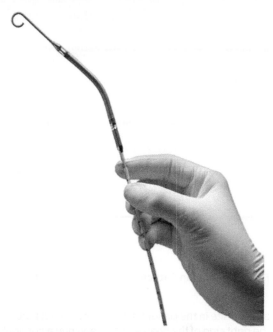

Fig. 1. The Impella cVAD has a 9-F shaft/14-F pump, allowing percutaneous insertion, and delivering up to 4 L/min support. (*Courtesy of* Abiomed Inc, Danvers, MA; with permission.)

chest wall and consists of a powerful, miniaturized pump with cannulae in the subclavian artery and vein through a transseptal approach capable of delivering up to 3 L per minute of support (**Fig. 4**). Such devices have been successfully implanted in animals and human studies are being planned.

The Mega 50-cc 8-F intra-aortic balloon (Maquet; Datascope Corp, Fairfield, NJ, USA) has just been made available and potentially adds more support than the 40-cc and 30-cc devices despite the same catheter shaft diameter.[32] The development of smaller, and portable pneumatic enhanced external counterpulsation devices has increased their potential for use in cardiogenic shock secondary to acute coronary syndromes.[33] The role of temporary LV stimulation through transjugular venous pacing in patients with deteriorating cardiogenic shock and evidence of LV dysynchrony represents another novel, less-invasive approach to providing circulatory support in such patients and early studies have been promising.[34]

Right Ventricular Support Devices

The Impella RP (right-side percutaneous; Abiomed). The US FDA has approved the use of the new right-sided percutaneous device in a forthcoming clinical study in the United States and there is some early clinical experience.[35] The Impella RP is a percutaneous heart pump that is implanted through a single

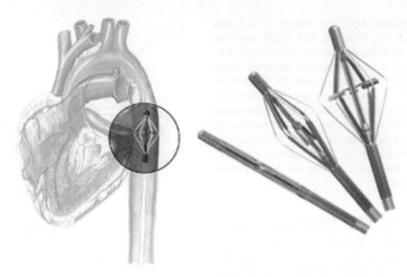

Fig. 2. The Reitan Catheter Pump. (*Courtesy of* CardioBridge GmbH, Hechingen, Germany; with permission.)

access site in the patient's leg and deployed across the right side of the heart without requiring a surgical procedure. The investigational device exemption enables the use of the Impella RP in a clinical study called RECOVER RIGHT. The study, which is expected to begin in early 2013, will enroll 30 patients from 10 different hospital sites and is estimated to take up to 24 months to complete. The study will enroll patients that present with signs of right-side heart failure, require hemodynamic support, and are being treated in the catheterization laboratory or cardiac surgery suite. The RECOVER RIGHT study will collect safety and effectiveness data on the percutaneous use of the Impella RP. Although the TandemHeart has been used in a large series of patients in the left ventricular assist device configuration, data on the use of this device as an RVAD have been reported if the catheters are positioned to pump right atrium to pulmonary artery instead

of the usual atrial-femoral circuit.[36,37] In the largest case series to date, 9 patients with refractory RV failure underwent percutaneous RVAD support with the TandemHeart. The average length of support was 3 days and resulted in significantly decreased right atrial pressure and increased mean arterial pressure, mixed venous saturation, and RV stroke work index.[38] The PulseCath iVAC 3L device has also been used for RV support for postcardiotomy RV failure.[39]

ECMO

Extracorporeal life support encompasses life support devices, including oxygenation, carbon dioxide removal, and hemodynamic support. Newer, minimized systems, such as the ELS-System and Cardiohelp (both from MAQUET Cardiopulmonary AG, Hirrlingen, Germany; **Fig. 5**), have been developed with smaller cannulae and

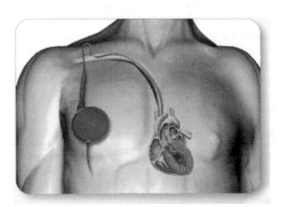

Fig. 3. The iVAC 3L device. (*Courtesy of* PulseCath BV, Amsterdam, the Netherlands; with permission.)

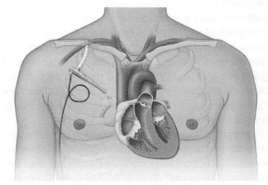

Fig. 4. The SYNERGY Micro-pump. (*Courtesy of* CircuLite, Inc, Saddle Brook, NJ; with permission.)

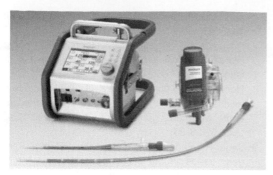

Fig. 5. The Cardiohelp portable ECMO system. (*Courtesy of* MAQUET Cardiopulmonary AG, Germany; with permission.)

hand-held devices, allowing rapid insertion and facilitated interhospital transport.[40,41]

Philipp and colleagues[41] used the portable Cardiohelp system for location-independent stabilization of 6 cardiopulmonary compromised patients with consecutive interhospital transfer and in-house treatment. The pre-ECMO ventilation time was 0.5 to 4 days and patients were transported by car or helicopter over a distance of 80 to 5850 km. The subsequent in-house ECMO support was continued with the Cardiohelp and lasted for 5 to 13 days and 100% survival was achieved. More recently, the results of the cardiac-RESCUE pilot study from Paris have been published.[42] This program was designed to overcome the frequent lack of availability of ECMO and staff trained in its use by providing extra-institutional salvage circulatory support team in pre-existing regional referral networks. 104 refractory cardiogenic shock cases were assessed and 87 consecutively eligible patients (mean age 46 ± 15 years, 41% following cardiac arrest) had ECMO support instituted locally and were enrolled into the program. Local initiation of ECMO support allowed successful transfer to the tertiary-care center in 75 patients. Of these, 32 patients survived to hospital discharge (overall survival rate 36.8%, 95% confidence interval [CI] 27.4–46.2). Independent predictors for in-hospital mortality included initiation of ECMO during cardiopulmonary resuscitation (hazard ratio [HR] = 4.81, 95% CI 2.25–10.30, $P<.001$) and oligo-anuria (HR = 2.48, 95% CI 1.29–4.76, $P = .006$). After adjusting for other confounding factors, in-hospital mortality was not statistically different from that of 123 consecutive patients who received ECMO at the host institution during the same period (odds ratio 1.48, 95% CI 0.72–3.00, $P = .29$). These data suggest that miniaturized ECMO systems can be used to stabilize and facilitate the transfer of greater than 80% of

referred shock patients, and that such a service seems feasible and potentially effective. Better identification of prognostic factors in shock patients could provide additional data to help refine indications; early independent predictors of in-hospital mortality included cause of the shock state, ECMO implantation during CPR, and severe liver or renal failure.

IMPROVEMENTS IN VASCULAR ACCESS MANAGEMENT

A reduction in vascular access point complications is essential for the increased uptake in pMCS devices, as such complications have an adverse effect on patient outcome and still arise in a significant proportion of patients in whom such devices are implanted.[43,44] Reducing catheter diameter size while maintaining sufficient device power is important in future device evolution. In addition, improved vascular closure techniques should be used. Many of these could be shared with closure techniques used in other interventional endovascular procedures, in particular, the rapidly developing field of transcatheter aortic valve implantation,[45,46] where experience, better patient selection, closure techniques, and reduction in device size has heralded a significant reduction in access site complications.[39] Devices, such as the Prostar percutaneous vascular device (Perclose Inc, Menlo Park, CA, USA), help maintain the minimally invasive approach and should be considered at the start of the procedure (preclosure technique),[40] avoiding the need for surgical cut-down. In patients with poor ileofemoral vessels, the alternative access sites can be considered and there is increasing experience using the Impella LP 5 device either via the axilllary artery[47,48] or insertion through a mini-sternotomy.[49]

THE EXPANDING ROLE OF PERIPHERAL MECHANICAL SUPPORT DEVICES

In addition to supporting patients with advanced heart failure and high-risk PCI, pMCS may have evolving roles in other areas of cardiology and beyond. Some data suggest that pMCS support may have a role in high-risk/unstable ventricular tachycardia catheter ablation procedures. The TandemHeart device was used for circulatory support during successful ventricular tachycardia ablation in a hypotensive patient.[50] Similarly, the Impella Recover 2.5 device was used for hemodynamic support in a series of patients during successful ablation of unstable ventricular tachycardia.[51] Of important note, the transseptal configuration of the TandemHeart catheter may potentially limit transseptal access for catheter ablation of ventricular tachycardia, and the presence of the Impella device within the LV cavity may also limit catheter movement. Both devices also limit groin access. Despite these potential physical challenges, the initial results mentioned above suggest the possibility of pMCS use as a bridge-to-electric-recovery device. After cardiac surgery, the Impella Recover 2.5 device has been shown to reduce mortality in postcardiotomy LV failure[43]; it has also been used in other specific situations such as hemostasis by left ventricular unloading, in a case with left ventricular posterior wall rupture,[52] and also for stabilization following acute ventricular septal defect complicating STEMI as a bridge to transplantation.[53] In other uses for pMCS beyond the heart and circulation, external counterpulsation has been suggested as a potential therapy for acute ischemic stroke by enhancing cerebral blood flow.[54]

SUMMARY

Although significant progress has been made in mechanical circulatory support over the last years, continued effort must be made to address this devastating clinical condition. Further research into appropriate patient selection, optimal timing of therapy, and novel device development must go hand in hand with the formation of collaborative circulatory support networks · involving both specialist and nonspecialist centers, with a focus on early referral and multidisciplinary discussion to try and improve patient outcomes, which still remain poor.

REFERENCES

1. French JK, Feldman HA, Assmann SF, et al. Influence of thrombolytic therapy, with or without intra-aortic balloon counterpulsation, on 12-month survival in the shock trial. Am Heart J 2003;146: 804–10.
2. Thiele H, Zeymer U, Neumann FJ, et al. Intraaortic balloon support for myocardial infarction with cardiogenic shock. N Engl J Med 2012;367:1287–96.
3. O'Connor CM, Rogers JG. Evidence for overturning the guidelines in cardiogenic shock. N Engl J Med 2012;367:1349–50.
4. Basra SS, Loyalka P, Kar B. Current status of percutaneous ventricular assist devices for cardiogenic shock. Curr Opin Cardiol 2011;26:548–54.
5. Mancini D, Lietz K. Selection of cardiac transplantation candidates in 2010. Circulation 2010;122: 173–83.
6. Rose EA, Gelijns AC, Moskowitz AJ, et al. Long-term use of a left ventricular assist device for end-stage heart failure. N Engl J Med 2001;345: 1435–43.
7. Reynolds HR, Hochman JS. Cardiogenic shock: current concepts and improving outcomes. Circulation 2008;117:686–97.
8. Hoefer D, Ruttmann E, Poelzl G, et al. Outcome evaluation of the bridge-to-bridge concept in patients with cardiogenic shock. Ann Thorac Surg 2006;82:28–33.
9. Jeger RV, Radovanovic D, Hunziker PR, et al. Ten-year trends in the incidence and treatment of cardiogenic shock. Ann Intern Med 2008;149: 618–26.
10. Haft JW, Pagani FD, Romano MA, et al. Short- and long-term survival of patients transferred to a tertiary care center on temporary extracorporeal circulatory support. Ann Thorac Surg 2009;88:711–7 [discussion: 717–8].
11. Mehra MR, Kobashigawa J, Starling R, et al. Listing criteria for heart transplantation: International society for heart and lung transplantation guidelines for the care of cardiac transplant candidates–2006. J Heart Lung Transplant 2006;25:1024–42.
12. Levy WC, Mozaffarian D, Linker DT, et al. The Seattle heart failure model: prediction of survival in heart failure. Circulation 2006;113:1424–33.
13. Kalogeropoulos AP, Georgiopoulou VV, Giamouzis G, et al. Utility of the Seattle heart failure model in patients with advanced heart failure. J Am Coll Cardiol 2009;53:334–42.
14. Gorodeski EZ, Chu EC, Chow CH, et al. Application of the Seattle heart failure model in ambulatory patients presented to an advanced heart failure therapeutics committee. Circ Heart Fail 2010;3:706–14.
15. Fonarow GC, Adams KF Jr, Abraham WT, et al. Risk stratification for in-hospital mortality in acutely decompensated heart failure: classification and regression tree analysis. JAMA 2005;293:572–80.
16. Stevenson LW, Pagani FD, Young JB, et al. INTERMACS profiles of advanced heart failure: the current picture. J Heart Lung Transplant 2009;28: 535–41.
17. Alba AC, Rao V, Ivanov J, et al. Usefulness of the INTERMACS scale to predict outcomes after mechanical assist device implantation. J Heart Lung Transplant 2009;28:827–33.
18. Slaughter MS, Pagani FD, Rogers JG, et al. Clinical management of continuous-flow left ventricular assist devices in advanced heart failure. J Heart Lung Transplant 2010;29:S1–39.
19. Kirklin JK, Naftel DC, Kormos RL, et al. Second INTERMACS annual report: more than 1,000 primary left ventricular assist device implants. J Heart Lung Transplant 2010;29:1–10.
20. Oz MC, Rose EA, Levin HR. Selection criteria for placement of left ventricular assist devices. Am Heart J 1995;129:173–7.

21. Rao V, Oz MC, Flannery MA, et al. Revised screening scale to predict survival after insertion of a left ventricular assist device. J Thorac Cardiovasc Surg 2003;125:855–62.

22. Lietz K, Long JW, Kfoury AG, et al. Outcomes of left ventricular assist device implantation as destination therapy in the post-rematch era: implications for patient selection. Circulation 2007;116:497–505.

23. Abraham WT, Adams KF, Fonarow GC, et al. In-hospital mortality in patients with acute decompensated heart failure requiring intravenous vasoactive medications: an analysis from the acute decompensated heart failure national registry (ADHERE). J Am Coll Cardiol 2005;46:57–64.

24. Fincke R, Hochman JS, Lowe AM, et al. Cardiac power is the strongest hemodynamic correlate of mortality in cardiogenic shock: a report from the shock trial registry. J Am Coll Cardiol 2004;44:340–8.

25. Torgersen C, Schmittinger CA, Wagner S, et al. Hemodynamic variables and mortality in cardiogenic shock: a retrospective cohort study. Crit Care 2009;13:R157.

26. Jakovljevic DG, George RS, Donovan G, et al. Comparison of cardiac power output and exercise performance in patients with left ventricular assist devices, explanted (recovered) patients, and those with moderate to severe heart failure. Am J Cardiol 2010;105:1780–5.

27. Dunser MW, Hasibeder WR. Sympathetic overstimulation during critical illness: adverse effects of adrenergic stress. J Intensive Care Med 2009;24:293–316.

28. Soroff HS, Cloutier CT, Birtwell WC, et al. External counterpulsation. Management cardiogenic shock after myocardial infarction. JAMA 1974;229:1441–50.

29. Tsao NW, Shih CM, Yeh JS, et al. Extracorporeal membrane oxygenation-assisted primary percutaneous coronary intervention may improve survival of patients with acute myocardial infarction complicated by profound cardiogenic shock. J Crit Care 2012;27:530.e1–11.

30. Smith EJ, Reitan O, Keeble T, et al. A first-in-man study of the Reitan catheter pump for circulatory support in patients undergoing high-risk percutaneous coronary intervention. Catheter Cardiovasc Interv 2009;73:859–65.

31. Amico A, Brigiani MS, Vallabini A, et al. Pulsecath, a new short-term ventricular assist device: our experience in off-pump coronary artery bypass graft surgery. J Cardiovasc Med (Hagerstown) 2008;9:423–6.

32. Mulholland J, Yarham G, Clements A, et al. Mechanical left ventricular support using a 50 cc 8 fr fibre-optic intra-aortic balloon technology: a case report. Perfusion 2013;28(2):109–13.

33. Cohen J, Grossman W, Michaels AD. Portable enhanced external counterpulsation for acute coronary syndrome and cardiogenic shock: a pilot study. Clin Cardiol 2007;30:223–8.

34. Eitel C, Gaspar T, Bode K, et al. Temporary left ventricular stimulation in patients with refractory cardiogenic shock and asynchronous left ventricular contraction: a safety and feasibility study. Heart Rhythm 2013;10(1):46–52.

35. Cheung A, Leprince P, Freed D. First clinical evaluation of a novel percutaneous right ventricular assist device: the impella rp. J Am Coll Cardiol 2012;59:E872.

36. Kar B, Gregoric ID, Basra SS, et al. The percutaneous ventricular assist device in severe refractory cardiogenic shock. J Am Coll Cardiol 2011;57:688–96.

37. Kar B, Adkins LE, Civitello AB, et al. Clinical experience with the TandemHeart percutaneous ventricular assist device. Tex Heart Inst J 2006;33:111–5.

38. Kapur NK, Paruchuri V, Korabathina R, et al. Effects of a percutaneous mechanical circulatory support device for medically refractory right ventricular failure. J Heart Lung Transplant 2011;30:1360–7.

39. Arrigoni SC, Kuijpers M, Mecozzi G, et al. Pulsecath(r) as a right ventricular assist device. Interact Cardiovasc Thorac Surg 2011;12:891–4.

40. Arlt M, Philipp A, Voelkel S, et al. Hand-held minimised extracorporeal membrane oxygenation: a new bridge to recovery in patients with out-of-centre cardiogenic shock. Eur J Cardiothorac Surg 2011;40:689–94.

41. Philipp A, Arlt M, Amann M, et al. First experience with the ultra compact mobile extracorporeal membrane oxygenation system Cardiohelp in interhospital transport. Interact Cardiovasc Thorac Surg 2011;12:978–81.

42. Beurtheret S, Mordant P, Paoletti X, et al. Emergency circulatory support in refractory cardiogenic shock patients in remote institutions: a pilot study (the cardiac-rescue program). Eur Heart J 2013;34:112–20.

43. Siegenthaler MP, Brehm K, Strecker T, et al. The Impella recover microaxial left ventricular assist device reduces mortality for postcardiotomy failure: a three-center experience. J Thorac Cardiovasc Surg 2004;127:812–22.

44. Cheng JM, den Uil CA, Hoeks SE, et al. Percutaneous left ventricular assist devices vs. Intra-aortic balloon pump counterpulsation for treatment of cardiogenic shock: a meta-analysis of controlled trials. Eur Heart J 2009;30:2102–8.

45. Cockburn J, De Belder A, Trivedi U, et al. Vascular closure after transcatheter aortic valve interventions–the current state of play. J Interv Cardiol 2012;25:526–32.

46. Cockburn J, de Belder A, Brooks M, et al. Large calibre arterial access device closure for percutaneous aortic valve interventions: use of the Prostar system in 118 cases. Catheter Cardiovasc Interv 2012;79:143–9.

47. Lam K, Sjauw KD, van der Meulen J, et al. A combined surgical and percutaneous approach through the axillary artery to introduce the Impella LP5.0 for short-term circulatory support. Int J Cardiol 2009;134:277–9.

48. Sassard T, Scalabre A, Bonnefoy E, et al. The right axillary artery approach for the Impella recover LP 5.0 microaxial pump. Ann Thorac Surg 2008;85: 1468–70.

49. Oses P, Casassus F, Leroux L, et al. Optimization of Impella 5.0 implantation using mini-sternotomy approach in postmyocardial infarction cardiogenic shock. J Cardiovasc Surg 2012;27:605–6.

50. Friedman PA, Munger TM, Torres N, et al. Percutaneous endocardial and epicardial ablation of hypotensive ventricular tachycardia with percutaneous left ventricular assist in the electrophysiology laboratory. J Cardiovasc Electrophysiol 2007;18:106–9.

51. Abuissa H, Roshan J, Lim B, et al. Use of the Impella microaxial blood pump for ablation of hemodynamically unstable ventricular tachycardia. J Cardiovasc Electrophysiol 2010;21:458–61.

52. Dahlin LG, Peterzen B. Impella used for hemostasis by left ventricular unloading, in a case with left ventricular posterior wall rupture. Ann Thorac Surg 2008;85:1445–7.

53. Patane F, Zingarelli E, Sansone F, et al. Acute ventricular septal defect treated with an Impella recovery as a 'bridge therapy' to heart transplantation. Interact Cardiovasc Thorac Surg 2007;6: 818–9.

54. Lin S, Liu M, Wu B, et al. External counterpulsation for acute ischaemic stroke. Cochrane Database Syst Rev 2012;(1):CD009264.

Index

Note: Page numbers of article titles are in **boldface** type.

A

Abiomed BVS System, for left ventricular cardiogenic shock, 460

Acute Decompensated Heart Failure National Registry, 488

Acute myocardial infarction
    cardiogenic shock in, **397–406**
    infarct size reduction in, **469–484**

Adenosine, for infarct size reduction, 472

Air embolism, in intra-arterial device therapy, 441

Amiodarone, for cardiac arrest, 432

Angioplasty, for infarct size reduction, 471

Anticoagulants, for cardiogenic shock, 400

Antiplatelet agents, for cardiogenic shock, 400

Aspirin, for cardiogenic shock, 400

B

Bio-Medicus device, for right ventricular failure, 449

Brain
    monitoring of, in cardiopulmonary resuscitation, 438
    perfusion of, in cardiopulmonary resuscitation, 440

C

Cardiac arrest, **429–443**
    cardiopulmonary support for, 433–434
    causes of, 431–432
    complications of, 440–441
    coronary ischemia causing, 430
    experimental, 435–438
    in severe cardiogenic shock, 434
    incidence of, 429
    left ventricular assist devices for, 433–441
    medical interventions for, 432–433
    outcomes of, 438–440
    prognosis for, 429–430, 432
    survival in, 430–431

Cardiac monitoring, in cardiopulmonary resuscitation, 438

Cardiac power output, 408, 472–473, 488

Cardiogenic shock, **397–406**
    clinical presentation of, 398
    etiology of, 398
    incidence of, 398

management of
    emergent, 400–402
    hemodynamic support for, 410
    in mechanical complications, 402–403
    innovative devices for, 403
    intra-aortic balloon pump for, 401, 458–460, 611
    left ventricular assist devices for, **457–468**
    medical, 399–400
    new devices for, **485–494**
    resuscitation in, 435
    revascularization for, 401–402
    stents for, 403
    strategies for, 398–399
    mortality in, 398–399
    pathophysiology of, 397–398, 457

CARDIOHELP system, 464, 490–491

Cardiopulmonary bypass, for cardiac arrest, 433

Cardiopulmonary resuscitation, **429–443**
    cardiopulmonary support in, 433–434
    cessation of, 440
    complications of, 440–441
    for cardiogenic shock, 434
    for coronary ischemia, 430
    for experimental cardiac arrest, 435–438
    incidence of, 429
    left ventricular devices for, 433–441
    medical interventions in, 432–433
    options for, 436, 438
    outcomes of, 438–440
    prognosis for, 429–430, 432

Cardiopulmonary support, for cardiac arrest, 433–434

CentriMag device
    for left ventricular cardiogenic shock, 460
    for right ventricular failure, 449, 453

Cerebral monitoring, in cardiopulmonary resuscitation, 438

Chain-of-survival, in cardiopulmonary resuscitation, 429

Compression devices, for cardiac arrest, 433

Coronary artery bypass graft surgery, for cardiogenic shock, 401–402

Coronary ischemia, cardiac arrest in, 430

Counterpulsation pump. *See* Intra-aortic balloon pump.

CRISP-AMI (Counterpulsation Reduces Infarct Size Pre-PCI) study, 474

Cyclosporine, for infarct size reduction, 472

Intervent Cardiol Clin 2 (2013) 495–498
http://dx.doi.org/10.1016/S2211-7458(13)00039-4

interventional.theclinics.com

Index

Printed and bound by CPI Group (UK) Ltd, Croydon, CR0 4YY

03/10/2024

01040346-0005